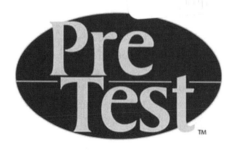

Clinical Vignettes for the USMLE Step 2 CK

PreTest™ Self-Assessment and Review

Notice

Medicine is an ever-changing science. As new research and clinical experience broaden our knowledge, changes in treatment and drug therapy are required. The authors and the publisher of this work have checked with sources believed to be reliable in their efforts to provide information that is complete and generally in accord with the standards accepted at the time of publication. However, in view of the possibility of human error or changes in medical sciences, neither the authors nor the publisher nor any other party who has been involved in the preparation or publication of this work warrants that the information contained herein is in every respect accurate or complete, and they disclaim all responsibility for any errors or omissions or for the results obtained from use of the information contained in this work. Readers are encouraged to confirm the information contained herein with other sources. For example and in particular, readers are advised to check the product information sheet included in the package of each drug they plan to administer to be certain that the information contained in this work is accurate and that changes have not been made in the recommended dose or in the contraindications for administration. This recommendation is of particular importance in connection with new or infrequently used drugs.

PreTest™

Clinical Vignettes for the USMLE Step 2 CK

PreTest™ Self-Assessment and Review

Fifth Edition

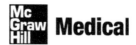

McGraw Hill Medical

New York   Chicago   San Francisco   Lisbon   London   Madrid   Mexico City
Milan   New Delhi   San Juan   Seoul   Singapore   Sydney   Toronto

The *McGraw·Hill* Companies

Clinical Vignettes for the USMLE Step 2 CK: PreTest™ Self-Assessm_
Fifth Edition

1 2 3 4 5 6 7 8 9 0   DOC/DOC   12 11 10 9

ISBN   978-0-07-160463-5
MHID 0-07-160463-4

This book was set in Berkeley by International Typesetting and Composition.
The editors were Kirsten Funk and Robert Pancotti.
The production supervisor was Sherri Souffrance.
Project management was provided by Madhu Bhardwaj, International Typesetting and Composition.
The cover designer was Maria Scharf.
RR Donnelley was printer and binder.

This book is printed on acid-free paper.

Library of Congress Cataloging-in-Publication Data

Clinical vignettes for the USMLE step 2 CK : PreTest™ self-assessment and review. —5th ed.
    p. ; cm.
  Includes bibliographical references.
  ISBN-13: 978-0-07-160463-5 (pbk. : alk. paper)
  ISBN-10: 0-07-160463-4 (pbk. : alk. paper)
    1. Medicine—Examinations, questions, etc.   2. Medicine—United States—Examinations, questions, etc.—Study guides.
  [DNLM: 1. Clinical Medicine—Examination Questions. WB 18.2 C64192   2009]
  R834.5.P676   2009
  610.76—dc22

                           2009007924

Contents

Preface

The current format of the United States Medical Licensing Examination Step 2 Clinical Knowledge (USMLE Step 2 CK) exam emphasizes clinical vignettes—-in single-best-answer multiple-choice and matching formats—as the primary test questions. The examination has approximately 370 multiple-choice questions, divided into eight blocks. Examinees have one hour to complete each block administered over a nine-hour testing session.

Clinical Vignettes for the USMLE Step 2 CK: Fifth Edition parallels this format. The book contains 368 clinical vignette-style questions covering the principles of clinical science and was assembled based on the published content outline for the USMLE Step 2. The questions are divided into eight blocks of 46 questions each. As on the Step 2 CK exam, each block tests the examinee on all core areas of clinical medicine. Answers are in the second half of the book. Each answer is accompanied by a concise but comprehensive explanation and is referenced to a key textbook or journal article for further reading.

The questions in this book were culled from the eight PreTest clinical science books. The publisher acknowledges and thanks the following authors for their contributions to this book:

Medicine: Robert S. Urban, MD, J. Rush Pierce, Jr, MD , Marjorie R. Jenkins, MD, Steven L. Berk, MD
Neurology: David J. Anschel, MD
Obstetrics and Gynecology: Karen M. Schneider, MD and Stephen K. Patrick, MD
Pediatrics: Robert J. Yetman, MD and Mark D. Hormann, MD
Psychiatry: Debra L. Klamen, MD and Philip Pan, MD
Surgery: Lillian S. Kao, MD and Tammy Lee, MD
Family Medicine: Doug Knutson, MD
Emergency Medicine: Adam J. Rosh, MD

McGraw-Hill
May 2009

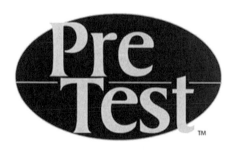

Clinical Vignettes for the USMLE Step 2 CK

PreTest™ Self-Assessment and Review

Block 1

Questions

1-1. A 59-year-old man presents to the ED with left-sided chest pain and shortness of breath that began 2 hours prior to arrival. He states the pain is pressure-like and radiates down his left arm. He is diaphoretic. His BP is 160/80 mm Hg, HR 86 beats per minute, and RR 15 breaths per minute. ECG reveals 2-mm ST-segment elevation in leads I, aVL, V_3 to V_6. Which of the following is an absolute contraindication to receiving thrombolytic therapy?

a. Systolic BP greater than 180 mm Hg
b. Patient on Coumadin and aspirin
c. Total hip replacement 3 months ago
d. Peptic ulcer disease
e. Previous hemorrhagic stroke

1-2. A 56-year-old woman is undergoing a cadaveric renal transplant. After revascularization of the transplanted kidney the transplanted renal parenchyma becomes swollen and blue. Which of the following statements is most accurate regarding her transplanted kidney?

a. The donor had preformed antibodies against the recipient's HLA antigens.
b. It is characterized pathologically by fibrin and platelet thrombosis of renal arterioles and small arteries and necrosis of the glomerular tufts.
c. Biopsies should not be obtained intraoperatively.
d. This form of rejection is associated with disseminated intravascular coagulation (DIC).
e. The rejection process can be treated with a steroid bolus and OKT3.

1-3. A 23-year-old woman comes to the psychiatrist because she "cannot get out of the shower." She tells the psychiatrist that she has been unable to go to her job as a secretary for the past 3 weeks because it takes her at least 4 hours to shower. She describes an elaborate ritual in which she must make sure that each part of her body has been scrubbed three times, in exactly the same order each time. She notes that her hands are raw and bloody from all the scrubbing. She states that she hates what she is doing to herself but becomes unbearably anxious each time she tries to stop. She notes that she has always taken long showers, but the problem has been worsening steadily for the past 5 months. She denies problems with friends or at work, other than the problems that currently are keeping her from going to work. Which of the following is the most likely diagnosis?

a. Attention-deficit hyperactivity disorder
b. Obsessive-compulsive disorder
c. Obsessive-compulsive personality disorder
d. Separation anxiety disorder
e. Brief psychotic disorder

1-4. A 30-year-old G1 with twin gestation at 28 weeks is being evaluated for vaginal bleeding and uterine contractions. A bedside ultrasound examination rules out the presence of a placenta previa. Fetal heart rate tracing is reactive on both twins, and the uterine contractions are every 2 to 3 minutes and last 60 seconds. A sterile speculum examination is negative for rupture membranes. A digital examination indicates that the cervix is 2 to 3 cm dilated and 50% effaced, and the presenting part is at −3 station. Tocolysis with magnesium sulfate is initiated and intravenous antibiotics are started for group B streptococcus prophylaxis. Betamethasone, a corticosteroid, is also administered. Which of the following statements regarding the use of betamethasone in the treatment of preterm labor is most accurate?

a. Betamethasone enhances the tocolytic effect of magnesium sulfate and decreases the risk of preterm delivery.
b. Betamethasone has been shown to decrease intraamniotic infections.
c. Betamethasone promotes fetal lung maturity and decreases the risk of respiratory distress syndrome.
d. The anti-inflammatory effect of betamethasone decreases the risk of GBS sepsis in the newborn.
e. Betamethasone is the only corticosteroid proven to cross the placenta.

1-5. A 35-year-old woman has noticed that over the past 3 to 5 months she has had some difficulties with balance, particularly when she closes her eyes. On examination, she has decreased hearing in her left ear and also left body dysdiadochokinesia. Her physician orders a head CT. Given this CT scan, which was obtained without contrast enhancement, the physician must assume that the posterior fossa mass at the arrow is which of the following?

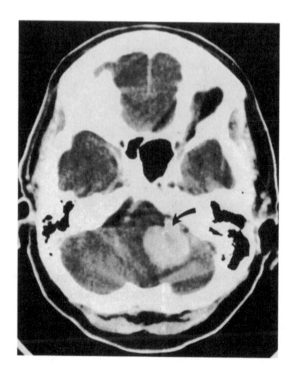

a. Normal
b. Calcified
c. Highly vascular
d. Granulomatous
e. Highly cystic

Questions 6 to 10

For each physical finding or group of findings, select the cardiovascular disorder with which it is most likely to be associated. Each lettered option may be used once, more than once, or not at all.

a. Massive tricuspid regurgitation
b. Aortic regurgitation
c. Coarctation of the aorta
d. Thoracic aortic aneurysm
e. Myocarditis

1-6. An elderly man with abnormal pupillary responses (Argyll Robertson pupil).

1-7. A 24-year-old drug addict with jugular venous distention and exophthalmos.

1-8. A patient with flushing and paling of the nail beds (Quincke pulse) and a bounding radial pulse.

1-9. A patient with conjunctivitis, urethral discharge, and arthralgia.

1-10. A patient with short stature, webbed neck, low-set ears, and epicanthal folds.

1-11. A 35-year-old previously healthy male develops cough with purulent sputum over several days. On presentation to the emergency room, he is lethargic. Temperature is 39°C, pulse 110, and blood pressure 100/70. He has rales and dullness to percussion at the left base. There is no rash. Flexion of the patient's neck when supine results in spontaneous flexion of hip and knee. Neurologic examination is otherwise normal. There is no papilledema. A lumbar puncture is performed in the emergency room. The cerebrospinal fluid (CSF) shows 8000 leukocytes/μL, 90% of which are polys. Glucose is 30 mg/dL with a peripheral glucose of 80 mg/dL. CSF protein is elevated to 200 mg/dL. A CSF Gram stain shows gram-positive diplococci. Which of the following is the best treatment option?

a. Begin acyclovir for herpes simplex encephalitis.
b. Obtain emergency MRI scan before beginning treatment.
c. Begin ceftriaxone and vancomycin for pneumococcal meningitis.
d. Begin ceftriaxone, vancomycin, and ampicillin to cover both pneumococci and *Listeria*.
e. Begin high-dose penicillin for meningococcal meningitis.

I-12. A 15-year-old girl is brought to the pediatric emergency room by the lunchroom teacher, who observed her sitting alone and crying. On questioning, the teacher learned that the girl had taken five unidentified tablets after having had an argument with her mother about a boyfriend of whom the mother disapproved. Toxicology studies are negative, and physical examination is normal. Which of the following is the most appropriate course of action?

a. Hospitalize the teenager on the adolescent ward.
b. Get a psychiatry consultation.
c. Get a social service consultation.
d. Arrange a family conference that includes the boyfriend.
e. Prescribe an antidepressant and arrange for a prompt clinic appointment.

I-13. A 22-year-old G1P0 at 28 weeks gestation by LMP presents to labor and delivery complaining of decreased fetal movement. She has had no prenatal care. On the fetal monitor there are no contractions. The fetal heart rate is 150 beats per minute and reactive. There are no decelerations in the fetal heart tracing. An ultrasound is performed in the radiology department and shows a 28-week fetus with normal-appearing anatomy and size consistent with dates. The placenta is implanted on the posterior uterine wall and its margin is well away from the cervix. A succenturiate lobe of the placenta is seen implanted low on the anterior wall of the uterus. Doppler flow studies indicate a blood vessel is traversing the cervix connecting the two lobes. This patient is most at risk for which of the following?

a. Premature rupture of the membranes
b. Fetal exsanguination after rupture of the membranes
c. Torsion of the umbilical cord caused by velamentous insertion of the umbilical cord
d. Amniotic fluid embolism
e. Placenta accreta

1-14. A 79-year-old man presents to the ED by paramedics with the chief complaint of agitation and confusion over the previous 12 hours. He has a past medical history of schizophrenia and is not taking any of his antipsychotics. His BP is 135/85 mm Hg, HR is 119 beats per minute, RR is 18 breaths per minute, oxygen saturation is 97% on room air, and fingerstick glucose is 135 mg/dL. Because of his agitation at triage, he was placed in wrist restraints. At this time, he is calm but confused. Examination reveals warm and clammy skin and 4-mm pupils that are equal and reactive. His cardiac examination reveals tachycardia and no murmurs. His lungs are clear to auscultation and his abdomen is soft and nontender. He is able to move all of his extremities. Which of the following is the most appropriate next step in management?

a. Administer haloperidol or lorazepam
b. Consult psychiatry
c. Order a CT scan of his head
d. Send a urine toxicologic screen
e. Obtain a rectal temperature

1-15. You are evaluating a 41-year-old man in your office who reports abdominal pain. He says the pain began suddenly and is located in the right lower quadrant. He describes the pain as "gnawing" and it seems to get worse after eating. He has vomited twice since the pain began. Which historical feature would lead you toward an emergent evaluation?

a. The pain's location in the right lower quadrant
b. The fact that the pain began suddenly
c. The description of the pain
d. The fact that it is worse after eating
e. The fact that it is associated with emesis

1-16. A 55-year-old man comes to the physician with the chief complaint of weight loss and a depressed mood. He feels tired all the time and is no longer interested in the normal activities he previously enjoyed. He feels quite apathetic overall. He has also noticed that he has frequent, nonspecific abdominal pain. Which of the following diagnoses needs to be ruled out for this man?

a. Pheochromocytoma
b. Pancreatic carcinoma
c. Adrenocortical insufficiency
d. Cushing syndrome
e. Huntington disease

I-17. A 39-year-old man presents to his physician with the complaint of loss of peripheral vision. Which of the following findings are demonstrated by the subsequent magnetic resonance imaging (MRI) scan, shown here?

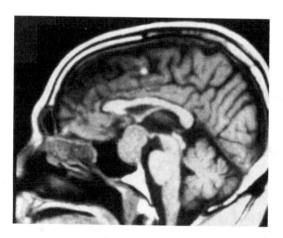

a. Cerebral atrophy
b. Pituitary adenoma
c. Optic glioma
d. Pontine hemorrhage
e. Multiple sclerosis plaque

I-18. A 16-year-old boy is struck on the side of the head by a bottle thrown by a friend involved in a prank. He appears dazed for about 30 seconds, but is apparently lucid for several minutes before he abruptly becomes stuporous. His limbs on the side opposite the site of the blow are more flaccid than those on the same side as the injury. On arrival in the emergency room 25 minutes after the accident, he is unresponsive to painful stimuli. His pulse is 40 beats per minute, with an ECG revealing no arrhythmias. His blood pressure in both arms is 170/110 mm Hg. Although papilledema is not evident in his fundi, he has venous distention and absent pulsations of the retinal vasculature. Which of the following is the best explanation for this young man's evolving clinical signs?

a. A seizure disorder
b. A cardiac conduction defect
c. Increased intracranial pressure
d. Sick sinus syndrome
e. Communicating hydrocephalus

1-19. A 30-year-old woman presents with hypertension, weakness, bone pain, and a serum calcium level of 15.2 mg/dL. Hand films below show osteitis fibrosa cystica. Which of the following is the most likely cause of these findings?

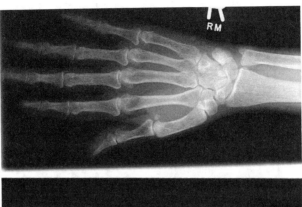

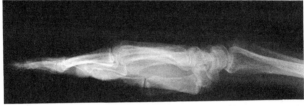

a. Sarcoidosis
b. Vitamin D intoxication
c. Paget disease
d. Metastatic carcinoma
e. Primary hyperparathyroidism

1-20. A healthy 9-month-old girl is brought to her pediatrician by her concerned parents. Previously very friendly with everyone, she now bursts into tears when she is approached by an unfamiliar adult. Which of the following best describes this child's behavior?

a. Separation anxiety
b. Insecure attachment
c. Simple phobia
d. Depressive position
e. Stranger anxiety

1-21. You are seeing a 78-year-old man who was brought to the office by his daughter. The daughter says her father is becoming increasingly forgetful. His medical history is significant for a 20-year history of type 2 diabetes and well-controlled hypertension. On examination, he is mildly hypertensive with otherwise normal vital signs. He is oriented to time, place, and person, but is unable to complete "serial sevens" on a mini-mental status examination. Which of the historical features make this diagnosis more consistent with dementia as opposed to delirium?

a. His history of hypertension
b. His history of diabetes
c. His current level of orientation
d. His inability to complete serial sevens
e. The recent onset of his symptoms

1-22. A 53-year-old woman is seeing you because of chronic nausea and vomiting. She has a 15-year history of type 2 diabetes mellitus. Her symptoms are worse after eating, and on occasion she will vomit food that appears to be undigested. Her weight is stable and she does not appear dehydrated. Which of the following is the best treatment for her condition?

a. An anticholinergic medication, like scopolamine (Transderm Scop)
b. An antihistamine, like promethazine (Phenergan)
c. A benzamide, like metoclopramide (Reglan)
d. A cannabinoid, like dronabinol (Marinol)
e. A phenothiazine, like chlorpromazine (Thorazine)

1-23. A 67-year-old man is brought to the ED by emergency medical service (EMS). His wife states that the patient was doing his usual chores around the house when all of a sudden he started complaining of severe abdominal pain. He has a past medical history of coronary artery disease and hypertension. His BP is 85/70 mm Hg, HR is 105 beats per minute, temperature is 98.9°F, and his RR is 18 breaths per minute. On physical examination, he is diaphoretic and in obvious pain. Upon palpating his abdomen, you feel a large pulsatile mass. An electrocardiogram (ECG) reveals sinus tachycardia. You place the patient on a monitor, administer oxygen, insert two large-bore IVs, and send his blood to the laboratory. His BP does not improve after a 1-L fluid bolus. Which of the following is the most appropriate next step in management?

a. Order a CT scan to evaluate his aorta.
b. Call the angiography suite and have them prepare the room for the patient.
c. Order a portable abdominal radiograph.
d. Call surgery and have them prepare the operating room (OR) for an exploratory laparotomy.
e. Call the cardiac catheterization laboratory to prepare for stent insertion.

1-24. A patient is seen on the first postoperative day after a difficult abdominal hysterectomy complicated by hemorrhage from the left uterine artery pedicle. Multiple sutures were placed into this area to control bleeding. Her estimated blood loss was 500 mL. The patient now has fever, left back pain, left costovertebral angle tenderness, and hematuria. Her vital signs are temperature 38.2°C (100.8°F), blood pressure 110/80 mm Hg, respiratory rate 18 breaths per minute, and pulse 102 beats per minute. Her postoperative hemoglobin dropped from 11.2 to 9.8, her white blood cell count is 9.5, and her creatinine rose from 0.6 mg/dL to 1.8 mg/dL. What is next best step in the management of this patient?

a. Order chest x-ray.
b. Order intravenous pyelogram.
c. Order renal ultrasound.
d. Start intravenous antibiotics.
e. Transfuse two units of packed red blood cells.

1-25. A 15-month-old boy is brought to the ER because of fever and a rash. Six hours earlier he was fine, except for tugging on his ears; another physician diagnosed otitis media and prescribed amoxicillin. During the interim period, the child has developed an erythematous rash on his face, trunk, and extremities. Some of the lesions, which are of variable size, do not blanch on pressure. The child is now very irritable, and he does not interact well with the examiner. Temperature is 39.5°C (103.1°F). He continues to have injected, immobile tympanic membranes, but you are concerned about his change in mental status. Which of the following is the most appropriate next step in the management of this infant?

a. Begin administration of IV ampicillin
b. Begin diphenhydramine
c. Discontinue administration of ampicillin and begin trimethoprim with sulfamethoxazole
d. Perform bilateral myringotomies
e. Perform a lumbar puncture

I-26. A 63-year-old painter complains of severe right shoulder pain. The pain is located posteriorly over the scapula. These symptoms began after he fell from a ladder 2 weeks ago. The pain is especially bad at night and makes it difficult for him to sleep. In addition, he has had some pain in the right upper arm. Treatment with acetaminophen and ibuprofen has been unsuccessful in controlling his pain. On examination the patient appears uncomfortable. The right shoulder has full range of motion. Movement of the shoulder is not painful. There is no tenderness to palpation of the scapula. What is the most likely diagnosis?

a. Subdeltoid bursitis
b. Rotator cuff tendonitis
c. Adhesive capsulitis
d. Osteoarthritis
e. Cervical radiculopathy

I-27. A 35-year-old woman complains of aching all over. She says she sleeps poorly and all her muscles and joints hurt. Her symptoms have progressed over several years. She reports she is desperate because pain and weakness often cause her to drop things. Physical examination shows multiple points of tenderness over the neck, shoulders, elbows, and wrists. There is no joint swelling or deformity. A complete blood count and erythrocyte sedimentation rate are normal. Rheumatoid factor is negative. Which of the following is the best therapeutic option in this patient?

a. Graded aerobic exercise
b. Prednisone
c. Weekly methotrexate
d. Hydroxychloroquine
e. A nonsteroidal antiinflammatory drug

I-28. A 26-year-old heroin addict has been using a street version of artificial heroin. The drug actually contains 1-methyl-4-phenyl-1,2,3,6-tetrahydropyridine (MPTP). The neurological syndrome for which he is at risk is clinically indistinguishable from which of the following?

a. Huntington disease
b. Friedreich disease
c. Sydenham chorea
d. Parkinson disease
e. Amyotrophic lateral sclerosis

1-29. You evaluate an 18-year-old male who sustained a right-sided cervical laceration during a gang fight. Your intern suggests nonoperative management and observation. Which of the following is a relative, rather than an absolute, indication for neck exploration?

a. Expanding hematoma
b. Dysphagia
c. Dysphonia
d. Pneumothorax
e. Hemoptysis

1-30. A 35-year-old woman is seeing a psychiatrist for treatment of her major depression. After 4 weeks on fluoxetine at 40 mg/day, her psychiatrist decides to try augmentation. Which of the following is the most appropriate medication?

a. Lithium
b. Sertraline
c. An MAO inhibitor
d. Clonazepam
e. Haloperidol

1-31. A recently retired 67-year-old woman presents to you to establish care. She was a long time smoker, but quit 5 years ago. She is generally healthy, but her prior physician told her that she has "emphysema." She was prescribed an "inhaler" to use as-needed and only uses it rarely. She asks about necessary immunizations. Assuming she has not had the vaccine before, which of the following vaccines should she receive?

a. MMR
b. Tdap
c. Varicella
d. Pneumococcal polysaccharide
e. Intranasal influenza

1-32. A 2-year-old child (A) presents with a 4-day history of a rash limited to the feet and ankles. The papular rash is both pruritic and erythematous. The 3-month-old sibling of this patient (B) has similar lesions also involving the head and neck. The most appropriate treatment for this condition includes which of the following?

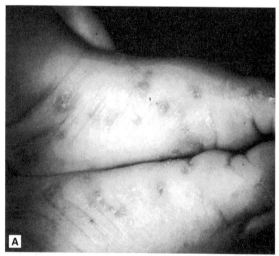

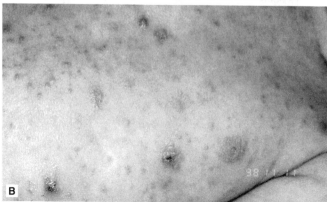

(Used with permission from Adelaide Hebert, MD.)

a. Coal-tar soap
b. Permethrin
c. Hydrocortisone cream
d. Emollients
e. Topical antifungal cream

1-33. A 70-year-old patient with chronic obstructive lung disease requires 2 L/min of nasal O_2 to treat his hypoxia, which is sometimes associated with angina. The patient develops pleuritic chest pain, fever, and purulent sputum. While using his oxygen at an increased flow of 5 L/min he becomes stuporous and develops a respiratory acidosis with CO_2 retention and worsening hypoxia. What would be the most appropriate next step in the management of this patient?

a. Stop oxygen.
b. Begin medroxyprogesterone.
c. Intubate and begin mechanical ventilation.
d. Observe patient 24 hours before changing therapy.
e. Begin sodium bicarbonate.

1-34. A 75-year-old G2P2 presents to your gynecology office for a routine examination. She tells you that she does not have an internist and does not remember the last time she had a physical examination. She says she is very healthy and denies taking any medication, including hormone replacement therapy. She has no history of abnormal Pap smears. She is a nonsmoker and has an occasional cocktail with her dinner. She does not have any complaints. In addition, she denies any family history of cancer. The patient tells you that she is a widow and lives alone in an apartment in town. Her grown children have families of their own and live far away. She states that she is self-sufficient and spends her time visiting friends and volunteering at a local museum. Her blood pressure is 140/70 mm Hg. Her height is 5 ft 4 in and she weighs 130 lb. Her physical examination is completely normal. Which of the following are the most appropriate screening tests to order for this patient?

a. Pap smear and mammogram
b. Pap smear, mammogram, and colonoscopy
c. Mammogram, colonoscopy, and bone densitometry
d. Mammogram, colonoscopy, bone densitometry, and TB skin test
e. Mammogram, colonoscopy, bone densitometry, TB skin test, and auditory testing

1-35. A 6-month-old girl is brought to the ED because of persistent crying for the past 6 hours. Her teenage father informs you that she has been inconsolable since awaking from her nap. No recent illness, trauma, fever, or other complaints are reported. On physical examination the patient is alert, awake, and crying. You note swelling, deformity, and tenderness of the left femur. When inquired about this finding, the caretaker responds, "Her leg got stuck between the rails of her crib." Radiographs show a minimally displaced spiral fracture of the left femur. Which of the following is the next best step in management?

a. Genetic workup for osteogenesis imperfecta and other bone abnormalities
b. Orthopedic consultation for closed reduction
c. Serum electrolytes including calcium and phosphate
d. Perform skeletal survey and contact Child Protective Services
e. Placement of posterior splint and discharge home with orthopedic follow-up

1-36. You are caring for a 45-year-old man with hypertension, gastroesophageal reflux, and depression. His medication list includes hydrochlorothiazide, verapamil, lisinopril, omeprazole, fluoxetine, and trazodone. He is complaining of difficulty with ejaculation. Which of the following medications is the most likely cause of this problem?

a. Hydrochlorothiazide
b. Verapamil
c. Lisinopril
d. Omeprazole
e. Fluoxetine

I-37. A 45-year-old woman with Crohn disease and a small intestinal fistula develops tetany during the second week of parenteral nutrition. The laboratory findings include:

Na: 135 mEq/L
K: 3.2 mEq/L
Cl: 103 mEq/L
HCO_3: 25 mEq/L
Ca: 8.2 mEq/L
Mg: 1.2 mEq/L
PO_4: 2.4 mEq/L
Albumin: 2.4

An arterial blood gas sample reveals a pH of 7.42, PCO_2 of 38 mm Hg, and PO_2 of 84 mm Hg. Which of the following is the most likely cause of the patient's tetany?

a. Hyperventilation
b. Hypocalcemia
c. Hypomagnesemia
d. Essential fatty acid deficiency
e. Focal seizure

I-38. A 23-year-old woman has 2 days of visual loss associated with discomfort in the right eye. She appears otherwise healthy, but her family reports recurrent problems with bladder control over the prior 2 years, which the patient is reluctant to discuss. On neurologic examination, this young woman exhibits dysmetria in her right arm, a plantar extensor response of the left foot, and slurred speech. Which of the following would be the most informative ancillary test?

a. Visual evoked response (VER) testing
b. Sural nerve biopsy
c. Electroencephalography (EEG)
d. Magnetic resonance imaging (MRI)
e. Computed tomography (CT)

1-39. A 32-year-old man living along the coast of Massachusetts presents with an acutely evolving left facial weakness. Although he has no facial pain or numbness, he does have a diffuse headache. He has no history of diabetes mellitus or other systemic illnesses, but does report newly appearing joint pains and a transient rash on his right leg that cleared spontaneously more than 1 month prior to the appearance of the facial weakness. On examination, he has mild neck stiffness and pain on hip flexion of the extended leg. This man is at highest risk for which of the following causes of a unilateral facial weakness?

a. HIV-associated neuropathy
b. Lyme neuropathy
c. Diphtheritic polyneuropathy
d. Tuberculous meningitis
e. Schwannoma

Questions 40 to 46

Match each type of delusional disorder with the vignette which best describes it. Each lettered option may be used once, more than once, or not at all.

a. Erotomanic
b. Grandiose
c. Jealous
d. Persecutory
e. Somatic
f. Mixed
g. Unspecified

1-40. A 48-year-old woman becomes convinced that her next door neighbor hates her and wants her to move. She states she has evidence, and when asked to explain, tells the psychiatrist that the neighbor gives her "looks," puts excessive junk in her mailbox, and leaves yard clippings on her side of the yard to harass her.

1-41. A 62-year-old man is arrested for disturbing people on their way to work by insisting they take his prepared reading materials with them. The topic of the materials was the man's special communications with God and his instructions for following him on a special path to heaven.

1-42. A 49-year-old man was arrested for beating up on his wife. He stated he had to punish her for having an affair—which she vehemently denied. The man's wife states to the police that the man has accused her of being interested in many other men over the course of their marriage. He now seems fixated on the topic.

1-43. A 39-year-old woman is arrested for breaking into the compound of a famous television star. She said she knew the star loved her and was giving her special messages to contact him from his weekly show.

1-44. A 19-year-old college student came to his primary care doctor for help with a foul odor he believed he was unintentionally emitting. The student stated that the odor left him socially isolated and that he was miserable about it. The primary care doctor could detect no odor.

1-45. A 22-year-old college student told his parents that on his plane ride home from college to see them over the holidays, all the seatmates on the plane had been replaced by aliens that were identical doubles to the humans that they had replaced.

1-46. A 58-year-old man called the police on his neighbors because he felt they were against him. When asked why, the man explained that the neighbors knew that he was a genius inventor, and they were unhappy about this because his impending fame would disrupt the neighborhood.

Block 2

Questions

2-1. A 75-year-old man goes out to shovel snow from his driveway. After 5 minutes of shoveling, he feels short of breath, chest pain, and then passes out. He awakens minutes later to his wife shaking him. In the ED, he denies chest pain or dyspnea. His BP is 160/85 mm Hg, HR is 71 beats per minute, and oxygen saturation is 97% on room air. On examination, you hear a harsh systolic ejection murmur. An ECG reveals a sinus rhythm with left ventricular hypertrophy. Which of the following is the most likely diagnosis?

a. Asystolic cardiac arrest
b. Brugada syndrome
c. Subclavian steal syndrome
d. PE
e. Aortic stenosis

2-2. A 31-year-old G3P3 Jehovah's Witness begins to bleed heavily 2 days after a cesarean section. She refuses transfusion and says that she would rather die than receive any blood or blood products. You personally feel that you cannot do nothing and watch her die. Appropriate actions that you can take under these circumstances include which of the following?

a. Telling the patient to find another physician who will care for her
b. Transfusing her forcibly
c. Letting her die, giving only supportive care
d. Getting a court order and transfusing
e. Having the patient's husband sign a release to forcibly transfuse her

2-3. At the time of delivery, a woman is noted to have a large volume of amniotic fluid. At 6 hours of age, her baby begins regurgitating small amounts of mucus and bile-stained fluid. Physical examination of the infant is normal, and an abdominal x-ray is obtained (see below). Which of the following is the most likely diagnosis of this infant's disorder?

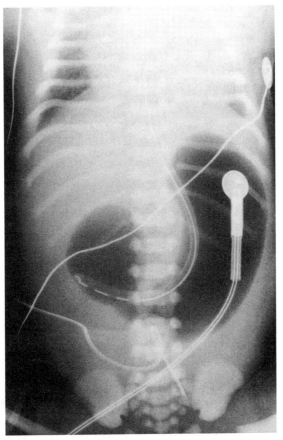

(Used with permission from Susan John, MD.)

a. Gastric duplication
b. Pyloric stenosis
c. Esophageal atresia
d. Duodenal atresia
e. Midgut volvulus

2-4. A 72-year-old man presents with progressive abdominal pain over the last 2 days. He has had several loose stools, subjective fever, and decreased appetite. Past medical history is significant for hypertension, diet-controlled diabetes mellitus, and one admission to the hospital for heart failure 2 years ago. He takes a beta-blocker and loop diuretic faithfully as prescribed by his physician. Vital signs include heart rate 92 and blood pressure 126/64. Physical examination reveals mucosal stranding of the oropharynx, no JVD, no lower extremity edema, and tenderness to palpation of the left lower quadrant of the abdomen. CT scan with contrast of the abdomen has been ordered. What is the best next step in the management of this patient?

a. Administer low-dose aspirin for prophylaxis of venous thromboembolism.
b. Administer low-dose low-molecular-weight heparin for prophylaxis of venous thromboembolism.
c. Administer treatment dose of low-molecular-weight heparin for presumed ischemic colitis.
d. Administer 600-mg N-acetylcysteine for prevention of contrast-induced nephropathy.
e. Administer 150-mEq sodium bicarbonate in 1-L D5 water for prevention of contrast-induced nephropathy.

2-5. A 72-year-old Caucasian male presents with shortness of breath that awakens him at night. At baseline he is able to walk less than a block before stopping to catch his breath. Physical examination findings include bilateral basilar rales and neck vein distention. The patient has a known history of congestive heart failure, and his last echocardiogram revealed an ejection fraction of 25%. The patient is compliant with a medication regimen including an ACE inhibitor, beta-blocker, and loop diuretic. Blood pressure is well controlled. What additional treatment should you begin next?

a. Spironolactone
b. Aspirin
c. Amlodipine
d. Warfarin
e. Hydralazine and isosorbide dinitrate

2-6. A 6-year-old boy is brought to your practice by his paternal grandmother for his first visit. She has recently received custody of him after his mother entered the penal system in another state; she does not have much information about him. You note that the child is short for his age, has downslanting palpebral fissures, ptosis, low-set and malformed ears, a broad and webbed neck, shield chest, and cryptorchidism. You hear a systolic ejection murmur in the pulmonic region. His grandmother reports that he does well in regular classes, but has been diagnosed with learning disabilities and receives speech therapy for language delay. His constellation of symptoms is suggestive of which of the following?

a. Noonan syndrome
b. Congenital hypothyroidism
c. Turner syndrome
d. Congenital rubella
e. Down syndrome

2-7. A 25-year-old woman sees a psychiatrist for a chief complaint of having a depressed mood for her "entire life." She begins psychotherapy and sees the physician once per week. After 3 months of therapy, she tells the psychiatrist that she is very afraid of him because he is "so angry all the time." She behaves as if this is true and that the psychiatrist will explode with rage at any minute. The psychiatrist is not normally seen as an angry person and is unaware of any anger toward the patient. Which of the following defense mechanisms is this patient likely displaying?

a. Distortion
b. Blocking
c. Isolation
d. Projection
e. Dissociation

2-8. A 24-year-old white male presents with a persistent headache for the past few months. The headache has been gradually worsening and not responding to over-the-counter medicines. He reports trouble with his peripheral vision which he noticed while driving. He takes no medications. He denies illicit drug use but has smoked one pack of cigarettes per day since the age of 18. Past history is significant for an episode of kidney stones last year. He tells you no treatment was needed as he passed the stones, and he was told to increase his fluid intake.

Family history is positive for diabetes in his mother and a brother (age 20) who has had kidney stones from too much calcium and a "low sugar problem." His father died of some type of tumor at age 40. Physical examination reveals a deficit in temporal fields of vision and a few subcutaneous lipomas. Laboratory results are as follows:

Calcium: 11.8 mg/dL (normal 8.5-10.5)
Cr: 1.1 mg/dL
Bun: 17 mg/dL
Glucose: 70 mg/dL
Prolactin: 220 μg/L (normal 0-20)
Intact parathormone: 90 pg/mL (normal 8-51)

You suspect a pituitary tumor and order an MRI which reveals a 0.7 cm pituitary mass. Based on this patient's presentation, which of the following is the most probable diagnosis?

a. Tension headache
b. Multiple endocrine neoplasia Type 1 (MEN 1)
c. Primary hyperparathyroidism
d. Multiple endocrine neoplasia Type 2A (MEN 2A)
e. Prolactinoma

2-9. You are caring for a 38-year-old man with metastatic cancer. He thoroughly understands his condition, and realizes that he has only a few months to live. He asks that you do not tell his wife about his prognosis, as "she won't be able to take it." The patient's wife sees you in the hallway and says, "tell me the truth . . . how is his condition?" Which of the following responses best reflects an ethically sound course of action?

a. Tell her the truth about the situation because she has a right to know.
b. Tell her the truth because you have the legal obligation to do so.
c. Consult the ethics committee to help you make the decision.
d. Do not tell the patient's wife, but inform her that you will not tell her husband about the conversation you've just had.
e. Do not tell the patient's wife, but make an effort to encourage an open dialogue between her and her husband.

2-10. A 60-year-old otherwise healthy woman presents to her physician with a 3-week history of severe headaches. A contrast CT scan reveals a small, circular, hypodense lesion with ringlike contrast enhancement. Which of the following is the most likely diagnosis?

a. Brain abscess
b. High-grade astrocytoma
c. Parenchymal hemorrhage
d. Metastatic lesion
e. Toxoplasmosis

2-11. You are seeing a 46-year-old man who reports 3 months of discomfort centered around his upper abdomen. It is associated with heartburn, frequent belching, bloating, and occasional nausea. What is the most likely result that will be found after workup for these symptoms?

a. Peptic ulcer disease
b. GERD
c. Gastric cancer
d. Gastroparesis
e. No cause is likely to be identified

2-12. An 81-year-old woman with a history of type 2 diabetes mellitus and atrial fibrillation presents with right body weakness and slurred speech. She realized that there was a problem on awakening in the morning, and her husband called EMS, who brought her to the emergency room. There are no word-finding difficulties, dysesthesia, or headaches. She is taking warfarin. Physical examination findings include blood pressure of 210/95 and irregularly irregular heartbeat. There is left-side neglect with slurred speech. There is a corticospinal pattern of weakness of the right body, with the face and upper extremity worse than the lower extremity. Routine chemistries and cell counts are normal. Her INR is 1.7. Computed tomography (CT) of the head reveals a large right-sided subdural hematoma. The intracranial material appearing most dense on CT is which of the following?

a. Blood clot
b. White matter
c. Gray matter
d. Cerebrospinal fluid (CSF)
e. Pia mater

2-13. In the patient in the above vignette, which of the following features would be indicative of a good prognosis with this disease?

a. Young onset
b. Withdrawn behavior
c. Poor support system
d. Family history of mood disorders
e. Neurologic signs and symptoms present

2-14. A 21-year-old woman presents to the ED with a superficial 2-cm-midforehead laceration sustained from a fall. You irrigate and close the wound. The patient is an aspiring actress and concerned about her long-term cosmetic outcome. She requests detailed wound-care instructions. Which of the following statements would be an appropriate wound care instruction to give?

a. Avoid direct sun exposure while the wound is healing.
b. The wound should not be washed until sutures are removed.
c. Sutures should be removed in 7 to 10 days.
d. Appearance of the scar at suture removal will be the final cosmetic outcome.
e. Good suturing technique and meticulous wound care guarantees no scar formation.

2-15. A 56-year-old right-handed woman who had breast cancer 1 year ago began having neurological problems about 1 week ago. She began experiencing nausea, vomiting, and numbness in the right hand and foot. Today she is experiencing crescendo pain in the left retroorbital area. Her headache is throbbing and positional, particularly when she tries to bend forward. The headache was intense in the morning, and at times it woke her up last night. On examination, the only deficits are loss of double simultaneous tactile stimulation and right lower facial droop when smiling. Which of the following is the most appropriate next action?

a. Administer intravenous prochlorperazine
b. Give the patient a prescription for zolmitriptan
c. Make a follow-up appointment for next month
d. Order an electroencephalogram to rule out seizures
e. Get a brain MRI

2-16. Two weeks after a viral syndrome, a 2-year-old child develops bruising and generalized petechiae, more prominent over the legs. No hepatosplenomegaly or lymph node enlargement is noted. The examination is otherwise unremarkable. Laboratory testing shows the patient to have a normal hemoglobin, hematocrit, and white blood cell (WBC) count and differential. The platelet count is 15,000/μL. Which of the following is the most likely diagnosis?

a. Von Willebrand disease (vWD)
b. Acute leukemia
c. Idiopathic (immune) thrombocytopenic purpura (ITP)
d. Aplastic anemia
e. Thrombotic thrombocytopenic purpura

2-17. You are seeing a 17-year-old girl who reports intense vaginal itching and urinary frequency. She has been sexually active for 6 months. On examination, you note frothy yellow-green discharge with bright red vaginal mucosa and red macules on the cervix. What is the saline preparation of the discharge most likely to show?

a. Sheets of epithelial cells "studded" with bacteria
b. "Moth-eaten" epithelial cells
c. Motile triangular organisms with long tails
d. Many white blood cells
e. Hyphae

2-18. A 40-year-old man had undergone genetic testing several years ago for an autosomal dominant condition, which had afflicted members of his maternal family for several generations. The testing revealed he has the defective gene and now believes he is showing signs of the disease including nonpurposeful movement of the extremities which are socially awkward and make daily activities more difficult. If this patient were to be exposed to L-dopa, which of the following would most likely be evoked?

a. Generalized seizures
b. Partial seizures
c. Intention tremor
d. Scanning speech
e. Writhing and jerking movements of the limbs

2-19. For the first 6 hours following a long and difficult surgical repair of a 7-cm abdominal aortic aneurysm, a 70-year-old man has a total urinary output of 25 mL since the operation. Which of the following is the most appropriate diagnostic test to evaluate the cause of his oliguria?

a. Renal scan
b. Aortogram
c. Left heart preload pressures
d. Urinary sodium concentration
e. Creatinine clearance

2-20. A 21-year-old girl presents to the ED complaining of diarrhea, abdominal cramps, fever, anorexia, and weight loss for 3 days. Her BP is 127/75 mm Hg, HR is 91 beats per minute, and temperature is 100.8°F. Her abdomen is soft and nontender without rebound or guarding. WBC is 9200/μL, β-hCG is negative, urinalysis is unremarkable, and stool is guaiac positive. She tells you that she has had this similar presentation four times over the past 2 months. Which of the following extraintestinal manifestations is associated with Crohn disease but not ulcerative colitis?

a. Ankylosing spondylitis
b. Erythema nodosum
c. Nephrolithiasis
d. Thromboembolic disease
e. Uveitis

2-21. A 64-year-old woman presents to the emergency room with flank pain and fever. She noted dysuria over the past 3 days. Blood and urine cultures are obtained, and she is started on intravenous ciprofloxacin. Six hours after admission, she becomes tachycardic and her blood pressure drops. Her intravenous fluid is NS at 100 mL/h. Her current blood pressure is 79/43 mm Hg, heart rate is 128/minute, respiratory rate is 26/minute and temperature is 39.2°C (102.5°F). She seems drowsy yet uncomfortable. Extremities are warm with trace edema. What is the best next course of action?

a. Administer IV hydrocortisone at stress dose.
b. Begin norepinephrine infusion and titrate to mean arterial pressure greater than 65 mm Hg.
c. Add vancomycin to her antibiotic regimen for improved gram positive coverage.
d. Administer a bolus of normal saline.
e. Place a central venous line to monitor central venous oxygen saturation.

2-22. A 49-year-old man comes to the doctor with high blood pressure and anxiety. Preferring to try something other than medication at first, the patient agrees to try another approach. He is attached to an apparatus that measures skin temperature and emits a tone proportional to the temperature. Which of the following techniques is being used with this patient?

a. Hypnosis
b. Progressive muscle relaxation
c. Autogenic techniques
d. Placebo
e. Biofeedback

2-23. A 21-year-old woman returns to your office for evaluation of an abnormal Pap smear. The Pap smear showed a squamous abnormality suggestive of a high-grade squamous intraepithelial lesion (HGSIL). Colposcopy confirms the presence of a cervical lesion consistent with severe cervical dysplasia (CIN III). Which of the following human papilloma virus (HPV) types is most often associated with this type of lesion?

a. HPV type 6
b. HPV type 11
c. HPV type 16
d. HPV type 42
e. HPV type 44

2-24. A 47-year-old man with a history of hypertension presents to the ED complaining of continuous left-sided chest pain that began while snorting cocaine 1 hour ago. The patient states he never experienced chest pain in the past when using cocaine. His BP is 170/90 mm Hg, HR is 101 beats per minute, RR is 18 breaths per minute, and oxygen saturation is 98% on room air. The patient states that the only medication he takes is alprazolam to "calm his nerves." Which of the following medications is contraindicated in this patient?

a. Metoprolol
b. Diltiazem
c. Aspirin
d. Lorazepam
e. Nitroglycerin

2-25. During a routine appointment to discuss an upper respiratory infection, you find that your 18-year-old female patient has become sexually active for the first time. According to current guidelines, when should you begin cervical cancer screening on this patient?

a. At the current time
b. At the age of 19
c. At the age of 20
d. At the age of 21
e. Cervical cancer screening is not recommended

2-26. You are asked to evaluate an infant born vaginally 3 hours previously to a mother whose only pregnancy complication was poorly controlled gestational diabetes. The nursing staff noticed that the infant was breathing abnormally. On examination, you find that the infant is cyanotic, has irregular, labored breathing, and has decreased breath sounds on the right side. You also note decreased tone in the right arm. You provide oxygen and order a stat portable chest radiograph, which is normal. Which of the following studies is most likely to confirm your diagnosis?

a. Nasal wash for viral culture
b. Fiberoptic bronchoscopy
c. Chest CT
d. Chest ultrasound
e. Induced sputum culture

2-27. A 65-year-old man has had disrupted cerebrospinal fluid flow for several years, secondary to a thoracic disk herniation. This abnormal physiological state has resulted in the formation of a cervical cystic lesion readily apparent on MRI. Examination of this patient might reveal which of the following abnormalities?

a. Third-nerve palsy
b. Calf atrophy
c. Charcot joints
d. Atrophy of the intrinsic hand muscles
e. Grasp reflexes

2-28. A 43-year-old man with a gangrenous gallbladder and gram-negative sepsis agrees to participate in a research study. An assay of tumor necrosis factor (TNF) is performed. Which of the following is the origin of this peptide?

a. Fibroblasts
b. Damaged vascular endothelial cells
c. Monocytes/macrophages
d. Activated T lymphocytes
e. Activated killer lymphocytes

2-29. A very concerned mother brings a 2-year-old child to your office because of two episodes of a brief, shrill cry followed by a prolonged expiration and apnea. You have been following this child in your practice since birth and know the child to be a product of a normal pregnancy and delivery, to be growing and developing normally, and to have no chronic medical problems. The first episode occurred immediately after the mother refused to give the child some juice; the child became cyanotic, unconscious, and had generalized clonic jerks. A few moments later the child awakened and had no residual effects. The most recent episode (identical in nature) occurred at the grocery store when the child's father refused to purchase a toy for her. Your physical examination reveals a delightful child without unexpected physical examination findings. Which of the following is the most likely diagnosis?

a. Seizure disorder
b. Drug ingestion
c. Hyperactivity with attention deficit
d. Pervasive development disorder
e. Breath-holding spell

2-30. A 22-year-old woman presents to the emergency room with an episode of acute painful loss of vision in the right eye. On examination, there is a right afferent pupillary defect and papillitis on funduscopic examination. She has no history of neurologic symptoms. An MRI shows a few foci of T2 signal increase in a periventricular distribution. Which of the following is the most appropriate treatment for presumed optic neuritis in this patient?

a. Oral prednisone
b. Intravenous methylprednisolone
c. Cyclophosphamide
d. Plasma exchange
e. Intravenous gamma globulin

2-31. An attractive and well-dressed 22-year-old woman is arrested for prostitution, but on being booked at the jail, she is found to actually be a male. The patient tells the consulting physician that he is a female trapped in a male body and he has felt that way since he was a child. He has been taking female hormones and is attempting to find a surgeon who would remove his male genitals and create a vagina. Which of the following is the most likely diagnosis?

a. Homosexuality
b. Gender identity disorder
c. Transvestic fetishism
d. Delusional disorder
e. Schizophrenia

2-32. A 35-year-old G3P3 presents to your office 3 weeks after an uncomplicated vaginal delivery. She has been successfully breast-feeding. She complains of chills and a fever to 38.3°C (101°F) at home. She states that she feels like she has flu, but denies any sick contacts. She has no medical problems or prior surgeries. The patient denies any medicine allergies. On examination she has a low-grade temperature of 38°C (100.4°F) and generally appears in no distress. Head, ear, throat, lung, cardiac, abdominal, and pelvic examinations are within normal limits. A triangular area of erythema is located in the upper outer quadrant of the left breast. The area is tender to palpation. No masses are felt and no axillary lymphadenopathy is noted. Which of the following is the best option for treatment of this patient?

a. Admission to the hospital for intravenous antibiotics
b. Antipyretic for symptomatic relief
c. Incision and drainage
d. Oral dicloxacillin for 7 to 10 days
e. Oral erythromycin for 7 to 10 days

2-33. You are evaluating a 28-year-old man who is concerned about depression. He reports increased irritability, depressed mood, decreased enjoyment from usual activities, and sleep and appetite disturbances for 6 weeks. He reports a history of alcohol use, and currently has 6 beers a day on the weekdays, with up to 12 on the weekends. Which of the following is the most appropriate next step in treating his depression?

a. Treat with a selective serotonin reuptake inhibitor (SSRI)
b. Treat with bupropion
c. Recommend detoxification and abstinence
d. Recommend detoxification and abstinence and start an SSRI
e. Recommend detoxification and abstinence and start bupropion

2-34. A 74-year-old woman is admitted with upper gastrointestinal (GI) bleeding. She is started on H_2 blockers, but experiences another bleeding episode. Endoscopy documents diffuse gastric ulcerations. Omeprazole is added to the H_2 antagonists as a therapeutic approach to the management of acute gastric and duodenal ulcers. Which of the following is the mechanism of action of omeprazole?

a. Blockage of the breakdown of mucosa-damaging metabolites of nonsteroidal antiinflammatory drugs (NSAIDs)
b. Provision of a direct cytoprotective effect
c. Buffering of gastric acids
d. Inhibition of parietal cell hydrogen potassium ATPase (adenosine triphosphatase)
e. Inhibition of gastrin release and parietal cell acid production

2-35. A 20-year-old woman is brought to the emergency room by her family because they have been unable to get her to eat or drink anything for the past 2 days. The patient, although awake, is completely unresponsive both vocally and nonverbally. She actively resists any attempt to be moved. Her family reports that during the previous 7 months she became increasingly withdrawn, socially isolated, and bizarre; often speaking to people no one else could see. Which of the following is the most likely diagnosis?

a. Schizoaffective disorder
b. Delusional disorder
c. Schizophreniform disorder
d. Catatonia
e. PCP intoxication

2-36. You are seeing a 45-year-old diabetic woman who reports bilateral lower extremity peripheral edema. In addition to diabetes, she has hypertension and depression. Which of the following medications is the likely cause of her edema?

a. Fluoxetine
b. Metformin
c. Rosiglitazone
d. Lisinopril
e. Hydrochlorothiazide

2-37. A 75-year-old man presents to the ED with a depressed level of consciousness. His wife is at the bedside and states he was stacking heavy boxes when he complained of a sudden intense headache. He subsequently sat down on the couch and progressively lost consciousness. She states that he had a headache the previous week that was also sudden but not as intense. He had gone to visit his primary-care physician who sent him to have a CT scan of the brain, which was normal. Over the course of the past week, he complained of intermittent pulsating headaches for which he took sumatriptan. In the ED, you intubate the patient and obtain the noncontrast head CT seen below. The scan is most consistent with which diagnosis?

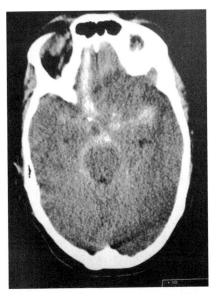

(Used with permission from Adam J Rosh, MD.)

a. Meningoencephalitis
b. SHA
c. Normal pressure hydrocephalus
d. Epidural hematoma
e. Subdural hematoma

2-38. The examination of a child's back is shown below. Evaluation with ultrasound of this lesion may demonstrate which of the following?

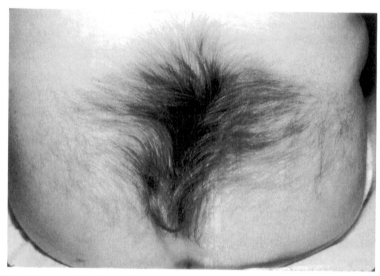

(Used with permission from Adelaide Hebert, MD.)

a. Epstein pearl
b. Mongolian spot
c. Cephalohematoma
d. Omphalocele
e. Occult spina bifida

Questions 39 to 41

For each clinical description, select the one most likely immunologic deficiency. Each lettered option may be used once, more than once, or not at all.

a. Wiskott-Aldrich syndrome
b. Ataxia telangiectasia
c. DiGeorge syndrome
d. Immunoglobulin A deficiency
e. Severe combined immunodeficiency
f. C1 inhibitor deficiency
g. Adenosine deaminase deficiency

2-39. A 16-year-old male has recurrent episodes of nonpruritic, nonerythematous angioedema. There is a family history of angioedema. The patient has also complained of recurring abdominal pain.

2-40. A 42-year-old man requires transfusion for blood loss resulting from an automobile accident. During the infusion, he develops urticaria, stridor, and hypotension requiring IV epinephrine. Further history reveals frequent episodes of sinusitis and bronchitis.

2-41. A 24-year-old female develops bronchiectasis after recurrent episodes of severe bronchitis and pneumonia. She has prominent blood vessels on the ocular sclera and across the bridge of the nose. Her sister had a similar illness and died of lymphoma at age 29.

Questions 42 to 46

Select the most probable diagnosis for each patient. Each lettered option may be used once, more than once, or not at all.

a. Churg Strauss syndrome
b. Cryoglobulinemic vasculitis
c. Temporal arteritis
d. Wegener granulomatosis
e. Takayasu arteritis
f. Polyarteritis nodosa
g. Henoch-Schönlein purpura

2-42. A 78-year-old man presents with a 2-month history of fever and intermittent abdominal pain. He develops peritoneal signs and at laparotomy is found to have an area of infarcted bowel. Biopsy shows inflammation of small- to medium-sized muscular arteries.

2-43. An elderly male presents with pain in his shoulders and hips. Temporal arteries are tender to palpation. ESR is 105 mm/L.

2-44. A 45-year-old man has wheezing for several weeks and now presents with severe tingling of the hands and feet. There is wasting of the intrinsic muscles of the hands and loss of sensation in the feet. WBC is 13,000 with 28% eosinophils.

2-45. A 42-year-old woman with hepatitis C develops fatigue, joint aches, and palpable purplish spots on her legs. Serum creatinine is 2.1 mg/dL and a 24-hour urine protein collection is 750 mg.

2-46. A 20-year-old female competitive swimmer notes that her arms now ache after swimming one or two laps, and she is unable to continue. She has had night sweats and a 10-lb weight loss. Pulses in the upper extremity are difficult to palpate.

Block 3

Questions

3-1. A 71-year-old woman presents to the ED after a reported mechanical fall 2 days ago. Her initial vitals include a HR of 55 beats per minute, a BP of 110/60 mm Hg, an RR of 14 breaths per minute, and an oxygen saturation of 96% on room air. The patient does not appear to be taking deep breaths. Her physical examination is significant for decreased breath sounds bilaterally and tenderness to palpation along the right side of her chest. After initial stabilization, which of the following is the diagnostic test of choice for this patient's condition?

a. Chest x-ray
b. Chest CT scan
c. ECG
d. Rib radiographs
e. Thoracentesis

3-2. A 72-year-old man undergoes an aortobifemoral graft for symptomatic aortoiliac occlusive disease. The inferior mesenteric artery (IMA) is ligated at its aortic attachment. Twenty-four hours after surgery the patient has abdominal distention, fever, and bloody diarrhea. Which of the following is the most appropriate diagnostic study for this patient?

a. Aortogram
b. Magnetic resonance imaging (MRI)
c. Computed tomographic (CT) scan
d. Sigmoidoscopy
e. Barium enema

3-3. A 55-day-old infant born prematurely at 27 weeks of gestation is shown below. The swelling is not tender, firm, hot, or red, and it does not transilluminate. It seems to resolve with pressure, but returns when the infant cries or strains. Which of the following is the most appropriate course of action at this point?

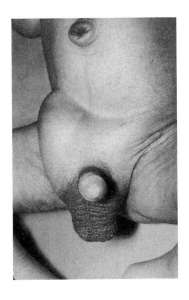

a. Obtain a surgical consultation
b. Perform a needle aspiration
c. Order a barium enema
d. Order a KUB (plain radiographs of kidney, ureter, and bladder)
e. Observe the patient and reassure the patient and family

3-4. Families of patients with schizophrenia, who are overtly hostile and overly controlling, affect the patient in which one of the following ways?

a. Increased relapse rate
b. Decreased rate of compliance
c. High likelihood that this behavior led to the patient's first break of the disease
d. Increased likelihood that the patient's schizophrenia will be of the paranoid type
e. Decreased risk of suicidal behavior

3-5. You are caring for a 19-year-old man who has been treated for mild intermittent asthma since childhood. He has been controlled using a short-acting bronchodilator as needed. Over the past month, he has been using his inhaler more than four times a week, and has had to wake up in the middle of the night to use his inhaler on three occasions. In the past, he was intolerant of the side-effects associated with an inhaled corticosteroid. Which of the following is the most appropriate treatment option?

a. Long-acting β-agonist
b. Leukotriene receptor antagonist
c. Cromolyn (Intal)
d. Theophylline
e. Oral corticosteroids

3-6. A 41-year-old man has had relapsing-remitting multiple sclerosis for nearly 20 years. Over that time his irreversible neurological deficits have gradually accumulated and he now has decreased visual acuity, poor coordination, and a spastic paraparesis. Cystometrographic analysis of bladder function in this patient is likely to show which of the following abnormalities?

a. Bladder hypotonia
b. Large residual volume of urine
c. Premature bladder emptying
d. Good voluntary control of bladder emptying
e. Urinary tract infection

3-7. A 25-year-old unhelmeted man involved in a motorcycle collision has multiple cerebral contusions on head computed tomographic (CT) scan. He is agitated but hemodynamically stable, with a heart rate of 80 beats per minute and a mean arterial pressure (MAP) of 90 mm Hg. An intracranial pressure monitor is placed, and the initial ICP reading is 30 mm Hg. Which of the following is the most appropriate in the management of his traumatic brain injury (TBI) over the next few days?

a. Hyperventilation to maintain a cerebral P_{CO_2} of 25 to 30 mm Hg
b. Administration of neosynephrine to increase his MAP and, consequently, his cerebral perfusion pressure (CPP)
c. Administration of mannitol (1 g/kg) to reduce his ICP
d. Placement of the patient in Trendelenburg position to increase cerebral perfusion
e. Avoidance of all sedating drugs in the first 24 to 48 hours in order to accurately assess his neurologic status

3-8. A 62-year-old man presents to the ED after he was found talking to himself by witnesses on a nearby street. Upon arrival, the patient appears confused and is actively hallucinating. His initial vitals include an irregular HR of 80 to 110 beats per minute, an RR of 14 breaths per minute, a BP of 160/80 mm Hg with an oxygen saturation of 97% on room air. An ECG indicates atrial fibrillation. The patient can be redirected but states that he is distracted by colorful, floating images in the room. Given this patient's presentation, what is the most likely etiology of his symptoms?

a. Acute psychotic disorder
b. Malingering
c. Conversion disorder
d. Digoxin overdose
e. Antidepressant overdose

3-9. A 25-year-old male presents to the clinic for evaluation of infertility. He has a life-long history of a productive cough and recurrent pulmonary infections. On his review of symptoms he has indicated chronic problems with abdominal pain, diarrhea, and difficulty gaining weight. He also has diabetes mellitus. His chest x-ray suggests bronchiectasis. Which is the most likely diagnosis?

a. COPD
b. Upper respiratory infections
c. Cystic fibrosis
d. Intrapulmonary hemorrhage
e. Asthma

3-10. An 85-year-old man is brought to the psychiatrist by his wife. She states that for the last 4 months, since the death of his son, the patient has been unable to sleep, has lost 20 lb, has crying spells, and in the last week has been starting to talk about suicide. She notes that he has numerous other medical problems, including prostatic hypertrophy, hypertension, insulin-dependent diabetes, and a history of myocardial infarction. Which of the following medications is most appropriate for the treatment of this patient?

a. Doxepin
b. Clonazepam
c. Sertraline
d. Tranylcypromine
e. Amitriptyline

3-11. You have been following a 15-month-old male infant. At 9 months, his height was at the 25th percentile while his weight was at the 5th percentile. At his 12-month visit, his weight and height are unchanged, so you asked his family to bring in a detailed dietary history and counseled them on a healthy diet. At his 15-month visit, his weight is up slightly, and his vital signs are as follows:

Blood pressure:	62/32 mm Hg (low)
Heart rate:	72 beats per minute
Respiratory rate:	16 breaths per minute
Temperature:	98.8°F

Which of the following is the best therapeutic option for this child?

a. Nutritional instruction to take two times the normal caloric intake
b. Iron supplementation with increased calorie intake
c. Zinc with increased caloric intake
d. Referral to social services for neglect
e. Hospital admission

3-12. A 71-year-old woman is brought to the emergency room by her daughter because of sudden onset of right-sided weakness and slurred speech. The patient, a recent immigrant from Southeast Asia, has not seen a doctor in 2 decades. Her symptoms began 75 minutes ago while she was eating breakfast. A stat noncontrast CT scan of the head is normal. Labs are normal. Physical examination reveals an anxious appearing woman with dense hemiplegia of the R upper and lower extremities. Deep tendon reflexes are not discernible on the R side and 2+ on the left. Aspirin has been given. What is the best next step in management of this patient?

a. Immediate intravenous unfractionated heparin
b. Immediate thrombolytic therapy
c. Immediate administration of interferon-beta
d. Emergent MRI/MRA of head
e. Emergent cardiac catheterization

3-13. A 10-year-old boy is admitted to the hospital because of bleeding. Pertinent laboratory findings include a platelet count of 50,000/μL, prothrombin time (PT) of 15 seconds (control 11.5 seconds), activated partial thromboplastin time (aPTT) of 51 seconds (control 36 seconds), thrombin time (TT) of 13.7 seconds (control 10.5 seconds), and factor VIII level of 14% (normal 38%-178%). Which of the following is the most likely cause of his bleeding?

a. Immune thrombocytopenic purpura (ITP)
b. Vitamin K deficiency
c. Disseminated intravascular coagulation (DIC)
d. Hemophilia A
e. Hemophilia B

3-14. A 17-year-old man presents to the ED with a lip laceration. He sustained the laceration during an altercation. On examination, he has a horizontal, 2-cm laceration of the right lower lip crossing the midline. There is significant swelling of the lower lip. The attending asks you, the intern, to perform a mental block for anesthesia. Which of the following statements regarding mental blocks is most accurate?

a. A mental block is performed by injecting lidocaine into the mental nerve foramen.
b. The patient requires a right-sided mental block.
c. A mental block is not appropriate in this patient because it will lead to worsened swelling of the lower lip swelling.
d. A mental block anesthetizes the mental nerve which innervates the lower lip.
e. A mental block is performed with a 3-cc syringe attached to an 18-gauge needle.

3-15. A 29-year-old woman has progressive gait disorder and dysmetria. Laboratory studies include a hematocrit of 55% and a routine urinalysis, which reveals excess protein and some RBCs in the urine. Urine culture is negative. The initial physical examination reveals an enlarged liver and spleen. Additional physical findings will most likely include which of the following?

a. A Kayser-Fleischer ring around the cornea
b. Hypopigmented (ash-leaf) spots on the trunk
c. Telangiectasias in the fundi on retinal examination
d. Bilateral hearing loss
e. Generalized hyporeflexia

3-16. A 16-year-old primigravida presents to your office at 35 weeks gestation. Her blood pressure is 170/110 mm Hg and she has 4+ proteinuria on a clean catch specimen of urine. She has significant swelling of her face and extremities. She denies having contractions. Her cervix is closed and uneffaced. The baby is breech by bedside ultrasonography. She says the baby's movements have decreased in the past 24 hours. Which of the following is the best next step in the management of this patient?

a. Send her to labor and delivery for a BPP.
b. Send her home with instructions to stay on strict bed rest until her swelling and blood pressure improve.
c. Admit her to the hospital for enforced bed rest and diuretic therapy to improve her swelling and blood pressure.
d. Admit her to the hospital for induction of labor.
e. Admit her to the hospital for cesarean delivery.

3-17. A 40-year-old school teacher develops nausea and vomiting at the beginning of the fall semester. Over the summer she had taught preschool children in a small town in Mexico. She is sexually active, but has not used intravenous drugs and has not received blood products. Physical examination reveals scleral icterus, right upper quadrant tenderness, and a palpable liver. Liver function tests show aspartate aminotransferase of 750 U/L (normal < 40) and alanine aminotransferase of 1020 U/L (normal < 45). The bilirubin is 13 mg/dL (normal < 1.4) and the alkaline phosphatase is normal. What further diagnostic test is most likely to be helpful?

a. Liver biopsy
b. Abdominal ultrasound
c. IgM antibody to hepatitis A
d. Antibody to hepatitis B surface antigen
e. Determination of hepatitis C RNA

3-18. A 55-year-old woman who has end-stage liver disease is referred to a hepatologist for evaluation. Which of the following would prevent her from being a transplantation candidate?

a. Use of alcohol 3 months ago
b. Two 2-cm hepatocellular carcinomas (HCCs) in the right lobe of the liver
c. A 4-cm hepatocellular carcinoma in the right lobe of the liver
d. Development of hepatorenal syndrome requiring hemodialysis
e. History of breast cancer 5 years ago with no evidence of disease currently

3-19. A 57-year-old woman began having weakness and trouble walking 1 year ago. Current examination findings include weak, wasted muscles with spasticity, fasciculations, extensor plantar responses, and hyperreflexia. Which of the following is the most likely diagnosis?

a. Dorsal spinal root disease
b. Ventral spinal root disease
c. Arcuate fasciculus damage
d. Motor neuron disease
e. Purkinje cell damage

3-20. You note that in your practice, a large number of women with a family history of breast cancer in a first-degree relative develop breast cancer themselves. You evaluate a number of charts, and find that 5% of the women in your practice who have breast cancer have a family history, but only 2% of women without breast cancer have a family history. Given this information, what is the sensitivity of using family history as a predictor of breast cancer in your patient population?

a. 2%
b. 5%
c. 93%
d. 95%
e. 98%

3-21. A 52-year-old man is sent to see a psychiatrist after he is disciplined at his job because he consistently turns in his assignments late. He insists that he is not about to turn in anything until it is "perfect, unlike all of my colleagues." He has few friends because he annoys them with his demands for "precise timeliness" and because of his lack of emotional warmth. This has been a lifelong pattern for the patient, though he refuses to believe the problems have anything to do with his personal behavior. Which of the following is the most likely diagnosis for this patient?

a. Obsessive-compulsive disorder
b. Obsessive-compulsive personality disorder
c. Borderline personality disorder
d. Bipolar disorder, mixed state
e. Anxiety disorder not otherwise specified

3-22. A 60-year-old woman with depression and poorly controlled type 2 diabetes mellitus complains of episodic vomiting over the last three months. She has constant nausea and early satiety. She vomits once or twice almost every day. In addition, she reports several months of mild abdominal discomfort that is localized to the upper abdomen and that sometimes awakens her at night. She has lost 5 lb of weight. Her diabetes has been poorly controlled (glycosylated hemoglobin recently was 9.5). Current medications are glyburide, metformin, and amitriptyline.

Her physical examination is normal except for mild abdominal distention and evidence of a peripheral sensory neuropathy. Complete blood count, serum electrolytes, BUN, creatinine, and liver function tests are all normal. Gallbladder sonogram is negative for gallstones. Upper GI series and CT scan of the abdomen are normal.

What is the best next step in the evaluation of this patient's symptoms?

a. Barium esophagram
b. Scintigraphic gastric emptying study
c. Colonoscopy
d. Liver biopsy
e. Small bowel biopsy

3-23. A 29-year-old woman presents to the ED complaining of double vision for 3 days. She states that she has been feeling very tired lately, particularly at the end of the day, when even her eyelids feel heavy. She feels better in the morning and after lunch when she is able to rest for an hour. Her BP is 132/75 mm Hg, HR is 70 beats per minute, temperature is 98.4°F, and RR is 12 breaths per minute. On examination you find ptosis and proximal muscle weakness. What is the most appropriate diagnostic test to perform?

a. Edrophonium test
b. Serologic testing for antibodies to acetylcholine receptors
c. Head computed tomography (CT) scan
d. Electrolyte panel
e. Lumbar puncture

3-24. A 22-year-old woman delivers a 7-lb male infant at 40 weeks without any complications. On day 3 of life, the infant develops respiratory distress, hypotension, tachycardia, listlessness, and oliguria. What is the most likely cause of the infant's illness?

a. Cytomegalovirus
b. Group B streptococcus
c. Hepatitis B
d. Herpes simplex
e. *L. monocytogenes*

3-25. A 25-year-old female with blonde hair and fair complexion complains of a mole on her upper back. The lesion is 8 mm in diameter, darkly pigmented, and asymmetric, with an irregular border (see illustration below). Which of the following is the best next step in management?

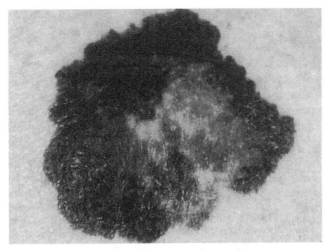

(Reproduced, with permission, from Fauci A et al. Harrison's Principles of Internal Medicine, 17th ed. New York, NY: McGraw-Hill, 2008.)

a. Tell the patient to avoid sunlight.
b. Follow the lesion for any evidence of growth.
c. Obtain metastatic workup.
d. Obtain full-thickness excisional biopsy.
e. Obtain shave biopsy.

3-26. Traditional therapies have offered limited benefit to a 55-year-old woman who suffers from migraine headaches, and she asks you about alternative therapies. She currently takes 325 mg of enteric-coated aspirin a day, and paroxetine, 20 mg daily. Which of the following has the lowest risk of toxicity or harm?

a. St. John's wort
b. Megavitamins
c. Macrobiotic diet
d. Ginkgo biloba
e. Acupuncture

Questions 27 to 31

For the most likely toxic substance involved in the cases below, select the appropriate treatment. Each lettered option may be used once, more than once, or not at all.

a. Atropine and pralidoxime (2-PAM)
b. *N*-acetylcysteine (Mucomyst)
c. Dimercaptosuccinic acid (DMSA, succimer)
d. Naloxone (Narcan)
e. Sodium bicarbonate

3-27. Over the past several weeks, a 2-year-old girl has exhibited developmental regression, abnormal sleep patterns, anorexia, irritability, and decreased activity. These symptoms have progressed to acute encephalopathy with vomiting, ataxia, and variable consciousness. The family recently moved, and they are in the process of restoring the interior of their home.

3-28. After a fight with her boyfriend, a 16-year-old girl took "some pills." At presentation she is alert and complains of emesis, diaphoresis, and malaise. Her initial liver function tests, obtained about 12-hour postingestion, are elevated. Repeat levels at 24-hours show markedly elevated aspartate aminotransferase (AST) and alanine aminotransferase (ALT), along with abnormal coagulation studies and an elevated bilirubin.

3-29. You are called to the delivery room. A newborn infant seems lethargic and has poor tone with only marginal respiratory effort, but his heart rate is above 100 beats per minute. The mother had an uncomplicated pregnancy, and delivery was uncomplicated and vaginal 10 minutes after spontaneous rupture of membranes. The mother received only pain medications while in labor.

3-30. A 4-year-old girl comes into the ER after eating a bottleful of small, chewable pills she found while at her grandfather's house. She has an increased respiratory rate, elevated temperature, vomiting, and is disoriented. She is intermittently complaining that "a bell is ringing" in her ears. She has a metabolic acidosis on an arterial blood gas.

3-31. After helping his father in the yard, a 14-year-old boy complains of weakness and feels like his muscles are twitching. He begins to drool, and then collapses in a generalized tonic-clonic seizure. Upon the arrival of EMS, his heart rate is found to be 40 beats per min and his pupils are pinpoint.

3-32. A 70-year-old woman undergoes a cardiac catheterization for exertional chest pain. Her pain continues to worsen and she is interested in having surgical treatment. Which of the following statements concerning CABG is most accurate?
a.   It is indicated for chronic and unstable angina.
b.   It is indicated for congestive heart failure.
c.   It is not indicated in patients with diabetes.
d.   It is associated with a 10% operative mortality in low-risk patients.
e.   It is indicated only if significant triple vessel disease is documented angiographically.

3-33. A 30-year-old man is brought to the emergency room after threatening to kill his 19-year-old girlfriend after she told him she was breaking up with him. The patient smells strongly of alcohol. The patient is from a high socioeconomic status and reports many social supports. Which of the following pairs of factors make this patient's risk of violent behavior higher?
a.   His age and his alcohol use
b.   His alcohol use and the impending breakup with the girlfriend
c.   The impending breakup with the girlfriend and his high socioeconomic status
d.   His high socioeconomic status and the presence of many social supports in his life
e.   The age difference of the couple and a verbal threat of violence by the patient

3-34. A 32-year-old man is brought into the ED by EMS with fever, shortness of breath, and stridor. The patient was treated yesterday in the ED for a viral syndrome. His BP is 90/50 mm Hg, HR is 110 beats per minute, temperature is 101.2°F, and his RR is 28 breaths per minute. A chest radiograph reveals a widened mediastinum. The patient is endotracheally intubated, given a 2-L bolus of normal saline, and started on antibiotics. His BP improves to 110/70 mm Hg and he is transferred to the intensive care unit (ICU). You see a friend that accompanied the patient to the hospital and ask him some questions. You find out that the patient is a drum maker and works with animal hides. What is the most likely organism that is responsible for the patient's presentation?

a. *Streptococcus pneumoniae*
b. *Corynebacterium diphtheriae*
c. *Coxiella burnetii*
d. *Haemophilus influenzae*
e. *Bacillus anthracis*

3-35. You are seeing a 19-year-old African American student who reports that he can "feel his heartbeat." It happens with exercise and is associated with some lightheadedness and shortness of breath. On examination, his heart has a regular rate and rhythm, but you hear a holosystolic murmur along his left sternal border. It increases with Valsalva maneuver. Which of the following is the most likely cause of his symptoms?

a. Mitral valve prolapse
b. Hypertrophic obstructive cardiomyopathy
c. Dilated cardiomyopathy
d. Atrial fibrillation
e. CHF

3-36. A 38-year-old man is seen by a psychiatrist because he has recurrent and intense sexually arousing fantasies involving wearing women's clothing. He notes that at first, he could wear women's underwear in his own home when he masturbated, and that this was sufficient. He now notes that he increasingly has the urge to wear women's clothes in public and masturbate somewhere less private. He comes in for help because he does not want to be caught at this behavior, though he is intensely attracted to it. He notes that he is a heterosexual, but that this cross-dressing behavior is sexually exciting to him. Which of the following disorders best describes this patient's symptoms?

a. Exhibitionism
b. Frotteurism
c. Sexual masochism
d. Transvestic fetishism
e. Gender identity disorder

3-37. A 52-year-old man with human immunodeficiency virus (HIV) and a history of intravenous drug use presents with a new heart murmur and fever. He also complains of severe back pain and on further evaluation is found to have an enlarged, saccular-appearing abdominal aorta below the renal arteries. Which of the following statements is correct regarding his diagnosis and treatment options?

a. The most likely organisms involved are *Staphylococcus* and *Salmonella*.
b. The mainstay of therapy should consist of antifungal antibiotics for 3 to 6 months.
c. Surgical intervention is indicated only if he remains febrile after 6 weeks of intravenous antibiotics.
d. The treatment of choice is aortic replacement with a synthetic graft and perioperative antibiotics only.
e. The treatment of choice is 6 weeks of intravenous antibiotics followed by aortic replacement with a synthetic graft.

3-38. An intravenous pyelogram (IVP) shows hydronephrosis in the workup of a patient with cervical cancer otherwise confined to a cervix of normal size. This indicates which one of the following stages?

a. Microinvasive stage
b. I
c. II
d. III

3-39. An 18-year-old woman is seeing you for an evaluation of her fatigue. She also complains of exercise intolerance and reports an unusual desire to chew ice in the last couple of months. You suspect anemia, and a point-of-care hemoglobin test confirms this diagnosis. What is the most likely cause of her anemia?

a. Iron deficiency
b. Lead toxicity
c. Autoimmune disease
d. Vitamin B_{12} deficiency
e. Folic acid deficiency

Questions 40 to 46

For each clinical scenario, select the most likely diagnosis. Each lettered option may be used once, more than once, or not at all.

a. Postictal state
b. Hypothyroidism
c. Uremic encephalopathy
d. Wernicke encephalopathy
e. Herpes encephalitis
f. Progressive multifocal leukoencephalopathy (PML)
g. Meningeal carcinomatosis
h. Central nervous system (CNS) toxoplasmosis
i. Multiple sclerosis
j. Hepatic encephalopathy
k. Subacute combined systems disease
l. Meningococcal meningitis
m. Subacute sclerosing panencephalitis (SSPE)
n. AIDS encephalopathy
o. Pickwickian syndrome

3-40. A 23-year-old woman with a history of hemophilia notices progressive memory difficulty. She has required little hematologic support, but she did receive transfusion of factor VIII at least five times over the past 7 years. Neurologic examination reveals word-finding difficulty, poor recent and remote memory, gait ataxia, mild dysarthria, and a labile affect. Her right plantar response is extensor and her left brachioradialis reflex is hyperactive with transient clonus. An MRI of the brain is unrevealing.

3-41. A 35-year-old businessman has sleep attacks. He runs a chain of dry-cleaning stores, but does not usually work with the cleaning fluids. He reports falling asleep several times during the workday, even at business meetings and during interviews. He has developed the sleep attacks only after gaining more than 100 lb. His weight at the time of the examination is 324 lb.

3-42. A 19-year-old man develops obvious personality changes over the course of 2 weeks. He becomes agitated with little provocation and abuses his wife both verbally and physically. His behavior is sufficiently atypical for it to prompt his relatives to seek psychiatric assistance for him. While being interviewed by a psychiatrist, he becomes unresponsive and develops generalized convulsions with opisthotonic posturing, tonic-clonic limb movements, and urinary incontinence. He is hospitalized for investigation of his seizure disorder. On initial examination, he is noted to have a low-grade fever and a mild left hemiparesis. His CSF opening pressure is 210 mm H_2O. His CSF cultures yield no growth, and his EEG reveals polyspike-and-wave discharges originating in the right temporal lobe. A CT of his brain reveals focal swelling of the right temporal lobe.

3-43. A previously healthy 25-year-old woman develops acute loss of vision in her left eye. She awakens with pain in the eye and reduction of her acuity to perception of light and dark. She delays seeing a physician for 1 week, during which time her acuity gradually improves sufficiently to allow her to read. On examination, the physician discovers she has slurred speech and poor rapid alternating movements with the left hand. Ocular dysmetria is evident in both eyes. Her tandem gait is grossly impaired. The physician obtains an EEG, which is normal.

3-44. A 17-year-old man has headache and photophobia on awakening. His physician discovers a low-grade fever and resistance to neck flexion. The physician advises the patient to take acetaminophen and remain in bed for the next 24 hours. Within 12 hours, the patient develops nausea and more intense headache. He seems disoriented and inappropriately lethargic. His family brings him to an emergency room. The emergency room physician notes a petechial rash on the legs and marked neck stiffness. CSF examination reveals a glucose content of 5 mg/dL, protein content of 87 mg/dL, and cell count of 112 leukocytes, with 70% polymorphonuclear cells.

3-45. A 56-year-old man is struck over the parietal area of the head during a robbery. He loses consciousness for 35 minutes but has no focal weakness or numbness on regaining consciousness. Within 2 days of the incident, his wife finds him unresponsive in bed early in the morning. She calls for an ambulance, but before it arrives her husband becomes more alert and asks for something to eat, saying he wants to have some supper before he goes to bed for the night. The ambulance attendant first on the scene notes that the patient is disoriented to place and time and has weakness of his right arm and leg.

3-46. A 35-year-old woman is found unconscious on the floor of her apartment. A bottle of cleaning fluid is found on a table near her. One of the contents indicated in the fluid is carbon tetrachloride. The ambulance crew notes that the patient is breathing independently, but her breath has a distinctly fetid odor unlike that associated with the cleaning fluid. Her limbs are flaccid, and she groans when she is moved. She does not respond to inquiries and is poorly responsive to pain. A serum ammonia level obtained at the emergency room is 250 mg/dL, triple the normal level. EEG reveals triphasic waves, most prominently over the front of the head.

Block 4

Questions

4-1. A 30-year-old G2P2 presents to the ED with acute onset of lower abdominal pain associated with vaginal bleeding that began 2 hours prior to arrival. She denies any prior medical history but does report having a tubal ligation after the birth of her second child. Her vitals are significant for a heart rate (HR) of 120 beats per minute and a blood pressure (BP) of 90/60 mm Hg. On physical examination, the patient has right adnexal tenderness with blood in the posterior vaginal vault. Her cervical os is closed. Given this patient's history and physical examination, which of the following is the most likely diagnosis?

a. Appendicitis
b. Pelvic inflammatory disease (PID)
c. Placenta previa
d. Ectopic pregnancy
e. Abruptio placentae

4-2. You are determining whether or not to use a rapid streptococcal antigen test to screen for streptococcal pharyngitis. You find that 2% of people with strep throat actually test negative using this test. Which of the following statements best describes this situation?

a. The sensitivity of the test is 2%.
b. The specificity of the test is 98%.
c. The test has a 2% false-negative rate.
d. The test has a 2% false-positive rate.
e. The test has a positive predictive value of 98%.

4-3. A 58-year-old postmenopausal female presents to your office on suggestion from a urologist. She has passed 3 kidney stones within the past 3 years. She is taking no medications. Her basic laboratory work shows the following:

Na: 139 mEq/L
K: 4.2 mEq/L
HCO_3: 25 mEq/L
Cl: 101 mEq/L
BUN: 19 mg/dL
Creatinine: 1.1 mg/dL
Ca: 11.2 mg/dL

A repeat calcium level is 11.4 mg/dL; PO_4 is 2.3 mmol/L (normal above 2.5). Which of the following tests will confirm the most likely diagnosis?

a. Serum ionized calcium
b. Thyroid function profile
c. Intact parathormone (iPTH) level
d. Liver function tests
e. 24-hour urine calcium

4-4. An 82-year-old previously healthy woman with a recent upper respiratory infection presents with generalized weakness, headache, and blurry vision. For the past 2 weeks she has had upper respiratory symptoms that started with a sore throat, nasal congestion, and excessive coughing. She went to her primary care doctor 4 days ago and was diagnosed with sinusitis. She was given a prescription for an antibiotic and took it for 2 days, then stopped. She thereafter had chills, lightheadedness, vomiting, blurry vision, general achiness, and a headache that started abruptly and has not gotten better since. Except for blurry vision, she has not had any other visual symptoms. The blurry vision remains when she closes either eye. She also has eye tenderness with movement and mild photosensitivity. She has no drug allergies. Examination findings include temperature of 102.5°F (39.16°C), nuchal rigidity, and sleepiness. Which of the following is the next most appropriate action in this case?

a. Get a brain MRI, then perform a lumbar puncture.
b. Give the patient a prescription for oral azithromycin and let her go home.
c. Immediately give intravenous ceftriaxone plus ampicillin.
d. Immediately start intravenous acyclovir.
e. Obtain CSF and blood cultures and observe the patient until the results come back.

4-5. A 15-year-old girl is seen in your clinic with a sprained ankle, which occurred the previous day while she was exercising in her room. You realize that you have not seen her for quite some time, and begin to expand your examination beyond the ankle. You find relatively minimal swelling on her right ankle. She has dental decay, especially of anterior teeth and a swollen, reddened, irritated uvula. She seems to be somewhat hirsute on her arms and legs, but has thinning of her hair of the head. She has a resting heart rate of 60 beats per minute, and her oral temperature is 35.5°C (96°F). Further questioning suggests that she has developed secondary amenorrhea. Which of the following is the most appropriate next step in the management of this girl?

a. Human immunodeficiency virus (HIV) testing
b. Radiograph of ankle
c. Thyroid function panel
d. Comparison of current and past weights
e. Pregnancy testing

4-6. After a prolonged fight with colon cancer, your 68-year-old patient decides to forego further attempts at curative treatment and focus on palliative care. He has tried nonsteroidal anti-inflammatory agents and acetaminophen for management of his pain, but this has been ineffective. Which of the following would be the best initial pain-management regimen?

a. A steroid burst to get the pain under control then scheduled nonsteroidal anti-inflammatory medications to maintain pain control
b. A long-acting narcotic pain patch at the lowest dose that controls the pain
c. A short-acting narcotic on a scheduled basis, with the possibility of additional short-acting narcotics as needed for breakthrough pain control
d. A long-acting narcotic, with a short-acting narcotic as needed for breakthrough pain
e. A patient-controlled analgesia device using opioids

4-7. A 50-year-old woman is diagnosed with cervical cancer. Which lymph node group would be the first involved in metastatic spread of this disease beyond the cervix and uterus?

a. Common iliac nodes
b. Parametrial nodes
c. External iliac nodes
d. Paracervical or ureteral nodes
e. Para-aortic nodes

4-8. You are asked to provide a 1-hour lecture to medical residents on the general topic of nutrition and cancer. You review a number of areas of interest. Which of the following statements concerning cancer and nutrition is correct?

a. Levels of nitrates in food and drinking water are positively correlated with the incidence of bladder cancer.
b. Regular ingestion of vitamin D from childhood probably inhibits formation of carcinogens.
c. Consumption of excessive amounts of animal dietary fats is associated with increased incidence of colon cancer.
d. Nutritional support of cancer patients improves response of the tumor to chemotherapy.
e. Alcohol ingestion is associated with pancreatic cancer.

4-9. A 58-year-old white man complains of intermittent rectal bleeding and, at the time of colonoscopy, is found to have internal hemorrhoids and the lesion shown at the splenic flexure. Pathology shows tubulovillous changes. Repeat colonoscopy should be recommended at what interval?

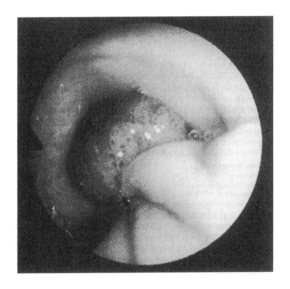

a. In 1 to 2 months
b. In 1 year
c. In 3 years
d. In 10 years
e. Repeat colonoscopy is not necessary

4-10. A 56-year-old woman who was diagnosed with paranoid schizophrenia in her early twenties has received daily doses of various typical neuroleptics for many years. For the past 2 years, she has had symptoms of tardive dyskinesia. Discontinuation of the neuroleptic is not possible because she becomes aggressive and violent in response to command hallucinations when she is not medicated. Which of the following actions should be taken next?

a. Start the patient on benztropine
b. Start the patient on amantadine
c. Start the patient on propranolol
d. Start the patient on diphenhydramine
e. Switch the patient to clozapine

4-11. A 37-year-old man has difficulty relaxing his grip on his golf club after putting. He also is excessively somnolent. Examination reveals early cataract development, testicular atrophy, and baldness. His family says that he has become increasingly stubborn and hostile over the past 3 years. His electrocardiogram (ECG) reveals a minor conduction defect. An electromyogram (EMG) will probably reveal which of the following?

a. Repetitive discharges with minor stimulation
b. Polyphasic giant action potentials
c. Fasciculations
d. Fibrillations
e. Positive waves

4-12. A 14-year-old boy presents with the complaint of "breast swelling." The boy reports that he has been in good health and without other problems, but has noticed over the past month or so that his left breast has been "achy" and that he has now noticed some mild swelling under the nipple. He has never seen discharge; the other breast has not been swelling; and he denies trauma. Your examination demonstrates a quarter-sized area of breast tissue under the left nipple that is not tender and has no discharge. The right breast has no such tissue. He has a normal genitourinary examination, and is Tanner stage 3. Which of the following is the best next course of action?

a. CT scan of the pituitary
b. Measurement of serum luteinizing hormone (LH) and follicle-stimulating hormone (FSH)
c. Measurement of serum testosterone
d. Reassurance of the normalcy of the condition
e. Chromosomes

4-13. A 26-year-old man presents to the ED in agony with a Gila monster still attached to his arm after being bitten. He reports that he is the animal's main handler, with no prior biting incidents. He reports localized pain but denies weakness, nausea, or feeling lightheaded. The animal bite occurred about 45 minutes ago. After the animal is carefully removed, what should be done next in the care of this patient?

a. Check for any remaining embedded teeth and begin wound care.
b. Administer antivenin.
c. Give tetanus prophylaxis.
d. Administer broad-spectrum antibiotics.
e. Apply suction device.

4-14. A 22-year-old has just been diagnosed with toxoplasmosis. You try to determine what her risk factors were. The highest risk association is which of the following?

a. Eating raw meat
b. Eating raw fish
c. Owning a dog
d. English nationality
e. Having viral infections in early pregnancy

4-15. A 5-year-old girl sustains a cut on her face from broken glass. Initially, the injury appears superficial except for a small area of deeper penetration just above the right eyebrow. Within 4 days, the child develops periorbital pain and double vision. The tissues about the eye are erythematous, and the eye appears to bulge slightly. The optic disc is sharp, and no afferent pupillary defect is apparent. Visual acuity in the affected eye is preserved. Which of the following is the most likely diagnosis?

a. Orbital cellulitis
b. Cavernous sinus thrombosis
c. Transverse sinus thrombosis
d. Optic neuritis
e. Diphtheritic polyneuropathy

4-16. You are seeing a patient who reports the abrupt onset of deep epigastric pain with radiation to the back associated with nausea, vomiting, sweating, and weakness. On examination, his abdomen is distended and tender in the epigastric area. Which of the following is the most common cause of this condition?

a. Gallstones
b. Alcohol abuse
c. Iatrogenic cause
d. Idiopathic cause
e. Hyperlipidemia

4-17. A 42-year-old woman presents to the ER with the worst headache of her life. A noncontrast CT scan of the head is negative for lesions or hemorrhage. She then undergoes a lumbar puncture, which appears bloody. All four tubes collected have red blood cell counts greater than 100,000/mL. Which of the following steps is the most appropriate management of this patient?

a. Repeat the head CT scan with intravenous contrast.
b. Perform an angiogram of the aorta and lumbar branches for immediate embolization of the injured vessel.
c. Perform a four-vessel cerebral angiogram.
d. Administer a dose of mannitol.
e. Consult neurosurgery for immediate ventriculostomy.

4-18. A 32-year-old woman presents to the ED after an aggressive outburst at work where her behavior was deemed a threat to others. Her coworkers state that she is normally very dependable, kind, and gracious but that over the course of the week they noticed that she was especially reserved and at times found her conversing with herself. Her initial vitals include HR of 89 beats per minute, RR of 15 breaths per minute, and BP of 130/75 mm Hg with oxygen saturation of 99% on room air. She tells you that she was recently started on a new medication. Which of the following types of medications may be responsible for this patient's behavior?

a. β-Blockers
b. Oral contraceptives
c. Corticosteroids
d. Nonsteroidal anti-inflammatory drugs (NSAIDs)
e. Calcium-channel blockers

4-19. A 40-year-old woman has had increasing fatigue and shortness of breath for years. Chest x-ray shows right ventricular hypertrophy and enlargement of the central pulmonary arteries. Pulmonary embolus is ruled out by spiral CT scan. Other causes of pulmonary hypertension have also been ruled out. Right heart catheterization reveals a pulmonary artery pressure of 75/30 mm Hg. Which of the following is the best next step in the management of the patient?

a. Acute drug testing with short-acting pulmonary vasodilators
b. High-dose nifedipine
c. Intravenous prostacyclin
d. Lung transplantation
e. Empiric trial of sildenafil

4-20. The parents of a 7-month-old boy arrive in your office with the child and a stack of medical records for a second opinion. The boy first started having problems after his circumcision in the nursery when he had prolonged bleeding. Studies were sent at the time for hemophilia, but factor VIII and IX activity were normal. At 2 months he developed bloody diarrhea, which his doctor assumed was a milk protein allergy and changed him to soy; his parents note he still has occasional bloody diarrhea. He has seen a dermatologist several times for eczema, and he has been admitted to the hospital twice for pneumococcal bacteremia. During both admissions, the parents were told that the infant's platelet count was low, but they have yet to attend the hematology appointment arranged for them. The child's WBC count and differential were normal. Which of the following is the most likely diagnosis in this child?

a. Idiopathic thrombocytopenic purpura
b. Wiskott-Aldrich syndrome
c. Acute lymphocytic leukemia
d. Adenosine deaminase deficiency
e. Partial thymic hypoplasia

4-21. A 43-year-old man has a father who died from Huntington disease. The son was tested and found to have the gene for Huntington disease. Which of the following is true regarding the offspring of those with Huntington disease?

a. Half the offspring are at risk only if the affected parent is male
b. Half the offspring are at risk only if the affected parent is female
c. Half the offspring are at risk if either parent is symptomatic for the disease before the age of 30
d. Half the offspring are at risk for the disease
e. One out of four children is at risk for the disease

4-22. You are evaluating a 26-year-old man with rectal pain. The pain was initially associated with bright red blood on the toilet paper after a bowel movement. Over the last day, his pain has worsened. On examination, he has an exquisitely tender purple nodule distal to the dentate line. Which of the following is the best treatment for his condition?

a. Hydrocortisone suppositories
b. Rubber band ligation
c. Sclerotherapy
d. Incision and drainage
e. Excision

4-23. A 20-year-old ataxic woman with a family history of Friedreich disease develops polyuria and excessive thirst over the course of a few weeks. She notices that she becomes fatigued easily and has intermittently blurred vision. Which of the following is the most likely explanation for her symptoms?

a. Inappropriate antidiuretic hormone
b. Diabetes mellitus
c. Panhypopituitarism
d. Progressive adrenal insufficiency
e. Hypothyroidism

4-24. A 28-year-old business executive sees her physician because she is having difficulty in her new position, as it requires her to do frequent public speaking. She states that she is terrified she will do or say something that will cause her extreme embarrassment. The patient says that when she must speak in public, she becomes extremely anxious and her heart beats uncontrollably. Based on this clinical picture, which of the following is the most likely diagnosis?

a. Panic disorder
b. Avoidant personality disorder
c. Specific phobia
d. Agoraphobia
e. Social phobia

4-25. A newborn has a midline defect in the anterior abdominal wall. The parents ask what, if anything, should be done. Spontaneous closure of which of the following congenital abnormalities of the abdominal wall generally occurs by the age of 4?

a. Umbilical hernia
b. Patent urachus
c. Patent omphalomesenteric duct
d. Omphalocele
e. Gastroschisis

4-26. You are seeing a 24-year-old woman who presents to your office complaining of "wheezing." She reports acute shortness of breath that occurred while she was shopping, and her wheezing is associated with pleuritic pain. She is otherwise healthy, only taking oral contraceptives. On examination, she is tachypneic, but not in acute distress. Auscultation of her lungs is normal. After the appropriate diagnostic workup, what is the best treatment option for this patient?

a. Reassurance and observation
b. Antibiotic therapy
c. Anticoagulation
d. Bronchodilators
e. Steroids

4-27. A 70-year-old female has been healthy except for hypertension treated with a thiazide diuretic. She presents with sudden onset of a severe, tearing chest pain, which radiates to the back and is associated with dyspnea and diaphoresis. Blood pressure is 210/94. Lung auscultation reveals bilateral basilar rales. A faint murmur of aortic insufficiency is heard. The BNP level is elevated at 550 pg/mL (Normal <100). ECG shows nonspecific ST-T changes. Chest x-ray suggests a widened mediastinum. Which of the following choices represents the best initial management?

a. IV furosemide plus IV loading dose of digoxin
b. Percutaneous coronary intervention with consideration of angioplasty and/or stenting
c. Blood cultures and rapid initiation of vancomycin plus gentamicin, followed by echocardiography
d. IV beta-blocker to control heart rate, IV nitroprusside to control blood pressure, transesophageal echocardiogram
e. IV heparin followed by CT pulmonary angiography

4-28. The family of a 4-year-old boy has just moved into your area. The child was recently brought to the emergency department (ED) for an evaluation of abdominal pain. Although appendicitis was ruled out in the ED and the child's abdominal pain has resolved, the ED physician requested that the family follow up in your office to evaluate an incidental finding of an elevated creatine kinase. The family notes that he was a late walker (began walking independently at about 18 months of age), that he is more clumsy than their daughter was at the same age (especially when trying to hold onto small objects), and that he seems to be somewhat sluggish when he runs, climbs stairs, rises from the ground after he sits, and rides his tricycle. A thorough history and physical examination are likely to reveal which of the following?

a. Hirsutism
b. Past seizure activity
c. Proximal muscle atrophy
d. Cataracts
e. Enlarged gonads

4-29. You are having trouble caring for a 58-year-old woman with uncontrolled diabetes. Her measures of glucose control are always significantly higher than you'd like to see, and you feel that she may not be taking her medications as directed. Which of the following is the most effective way to measure her adherence to the prescribed medical regimen?

a. Ask her if she is taking her medications.
b. Look for a reduction in her blood glucose measurements in subsequent visits.
c. Have her bring in her medications so that you may perform pill counts.
d. Measure serum blood levels of her medications.
e. Ask her specific questions about her medication names, dosages, and administration times.

4-30. A 40-year-old woman cut her finger while cooking in her kitchen. Two days later she became rapidly ill with fever and shaking chills. Her hand became painful and mildly erythematous. Later that evening her condition deteriorated as the erythema progressed and the hand became a dusky red. Bullae and decreased sensation to touch developed over the involved hand. What is the most important next step in the management of this patient?

a. Surgical consultation and exploration of the wound
b. Treatment with clindamycin for mixed aerobic-anaerobic infection
c. Treatment with penicillin for clostridia infection
d. Vancomycin to cover community-acquired methicillin-resistant *Staphylococcus*
e. Evaluation for acute osteomyelitis

4-31. A patient presents for her first initial OB visit after performing a home pregnancy test and gives a last menstrual period of about 8 weeks ago. She says she is not entirely sure of her dates, however, because she has a long history of irregular menses. Which of the following is the most accurate way of dating the pregnancy?

a. Determination of uterine size on pelvic examination
b. Quantitative serum human chorionic gonadotropin (HCG) level
c. Crown-rump length on abdominal or vaginal ultrasound
d. Determination of progesterone level along with serum HCG level
e. Quantification of a serum estradiol level

4-32. A 3-year-old African American boy with a history of sickle-cell disease presents to the ED after he developed a low-grade fever, runny nose, and an erythematous discoloration of both cheeks. His vital signs are heart rate (HR) 110 beats per minute, respiratory rate (RR) of 24 breaths per minute, and pulse oximetry of 98% on room air. The patient looks well and is in no acute distress. You note a macular lesion in both cheeks. The rash is not pruritic and there is no associated cellulitis or suppuration. What is the most serious complication to consider in this patient?

a. Osteomyelitis
b. Viral encephalitis
c. Pneumonia
d. Aplastic anemia
e. Meningitis

4-33. A biopsy is obtained from a clinically affected muscle in a person with several months of progressive weakness. The pathologist reports that there are numerous abnormally small muscle fibers intermingled with hypertrophied muscle fibers. The normal mosaic of muscle fiber types is disrupted. There is no significant inflammatory infiltrate. This pathologic description is most consistent with which of the following?

a. Disuse atrophy
b. Denervation atrophy
c. Muscular dystrophy
d. Polymyositis
e. Hypoxic damage

4-34. A 54-year-old man sees you because of a growth on his lip. He works in construction and is usually outdoors. The biopsy report confirms squamous cell carcinoma. Which of the following is most accurate in regard to this carcinoma?

a. The lesion often arises in areas of persistent hyperkeratosis.
b. More than 90% of cases occur on the upper lip.
c. The lesion constitutes 30% of all cancers of the oral cavity.
d. Radiotherapy is considered inappropriate treatment for these lesions.
e. Initial metastases are to the ipsilateral posterior cervical lymph nodes.

4-35. A 38-year-old obese female with history of chronic venous insufficiency and peripheral edema was admitted to the hospital the previous night for cellulitis involving both lower legs. She has had recurrent such episodes, treated successfully in the past with various antibiotics, including cefazolin, nafcillin, ampicillin/sulbactam, and levofloxacin. Intravenous levofloxacin was again chosen due to the perceived ease in transitioning to a once-daily oral outpatient dose. Normal saline at 50 mL/h is administered. Past history is otherwise significant only for hypertension, which is being treated at home with HCTZ 25 mg, lisinopril 40 mg, and atenolol 100 mg, all once each morning. Admission BP was 144/92 and the orders were written to continue each of these antihypertensives at one tablet po qd. The only other inhospital medication is daily prophylactic enoxaparin. As you round at 6 PM on the day following admission, the nurse contacts you emergently stating that she has just finished giving evening medicines and the patient's BP is unexpectedly 90/50. Pulse rate is 92. There is no chest pain, dyspnea, or tachypnea. What is most likely cause of her hypertension?

a. An allergic reaction either to the antibiotic or to one of the antihypertensives
b. A vasovagal reaction secondary to pain
c. Hypovolemia due to the cellulitis
d. Acute pulmonary embolism
e. Medication error

Questions 36 to 39

For each disorder listed below, select the peripheral blood smear with which it is most likely to be associated. Each lettered option may be used once, more than once, or not at all.

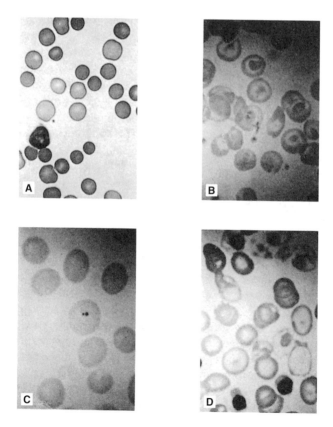

4-36. An 8-year-old patient with sickle-cell anemia

4-37. A 7-month-old boy with severe anemia requiring transfusions, heart failure, hepatosplenomegaly, and weakness

4-38. A 3-day-old newborn with anemia and pathologic hyperbilirubinemia requiring phototherapy

4-39. A completely asymptomatic, healthy 1-year-old whose routine CBC reveals an abnormality

Questions 40 to 46

Match the correct defense mechanism with each patient's actions. Each lettered option may be used once, more than once, or not at all.

a. Distortion
b. Repression
c. Reaction formation
d. Sublimation
e. Somatization
f. Intellectualization
g. Suppression
h. Isolation of affect
i. Introjection
j. Projection
k. Identification with the aggressor
l. Projective identification
m. Denial
n. Displacement

4-40. A patient starts complaining of chest pain and coughing whenever her therapist confronts her. She insists, however, that she is not at all distressed or angry.

4-41. A woman feels jealous and hurt when, at a family gathering, her husband flirts with her younger cousin. She makes a conscious decision to put her feelings aside and to wait for a more appropriate moment to confront her husband and convey her emotions.

4-42. A young man gets into an argument with his teacher. Although he is very upset, he remains silent as she chastises him severely and calls him a failure as a student. Once he gets home from school, the young man picks a fight with his younger brother over nothing and begins screaming at him.

4-43. A 34-year-old man is deeply envious of his younger but much more successful brother. Although it is difficult for him to admit, he believes the younger brother was their parents' favorite as well. He tells his friends that his younger brother is envious of his good looks and successes with women, even though there is some evidence that this is not so.

4-44. A 28-year-old woman is in psychotherapy for a long-standing depressed mood and poor self-esteem. One day during the session, the therapist yawns because she is very tired, though she is interested in what the patient has to say. The patient immediately bursts into tears, saying that the therapist must be bored and uninterested in her and must have been so for quite some time.

4-45. A man who, as a child, was beaten by his parents for every small infraction nonetheless idealizes them and describes them as "good parents who did not spoil their children." He is baffled and angry when he is ordered to start parenting classes after the school nurse reports that his children consistently come to school with bruises.

4-46. A 52-year-old man is hospitalized after a severe myocardial infarction. On the second day in the hospital, when his physician comes by on rounds, the patient insists on jumping out of bed and doing several push-ups to show the physician that "they can't keep a good man down—there is nothing wrong with me!"

Block 5

Questions

5-1. A 65-year-old black female presents for an annual examination. Physical examination is unremarkable for her age. In completing the appropriate screening tests you order a dual x-ray absorptiometry (DXA) to evaluate whether the patient has osteoporosis. DXA results reveal a T-score of −3.0 at the total hip and −2.7 at the spine, consistent with a diagnosis of osteoporosis. Since her Z-score is −2.0, you proceed with an initial evaluation of secondary osteoporosis. Laboratory evaluation reveals:

Calcium: 9.7 mg/dL
Cr: 1.0 mg/dL
Bun: 19 mg/d
Glucose: 98 mg/dL
25,OH vitamin D: 12 ng/mL (optimal >25)
WBC: 7700/μL
Hg: 12 g/dL
HCT: 38 g/dL
PLT: 255,000/μL

Based on the above information, additional laboratory would most likely reveal which of the following?

a. Elevated iPTH (intact parathormone), low ionized calcium, normal alkaline phosphatase
b. Normal iPTH, normal ionized calcium, elevated alkaline phosphatase
c. Elevated iPTH, normal ionized calcium, elevated alkaline phosphatase
d. Normal iPTH, low ionized calcium, elevated alkaline phosphatase
e. Elevated iPTH, low ionized calcium, normal alkaline phosphatase

5-2. You have diagnosed a 35-year-old African American man with hypertension. Lifestyle modifications helped reduce his blood pressure, but he was still above goal. You chose to start hydrochlorothiazide, 25 mg daily. This helped his blood pressure, but it is still 142/94 mm Hg. Which of the following is the best approach to take in this situation?

a. Increase his hydrochlorothiazide to 50 mg/d
b. Change to a loop diuretic
c. Change to an ACE inhibitor
d. Change to a β-blocker
e. Add an ACE inhibitor

5-3. A 29-year-old construction worker fell 15 ft from a roof and broke his right humerus, as depicted in the accompanying radiograph. Given his injury, which of the following nerves is most at risk?

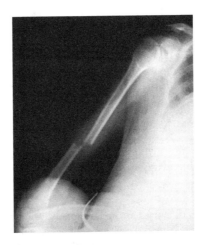

a. Median nerve
b. Radial nerve
c. Posterior interosseous nerve
d. Ulnar nerve
e. Ascending circumflex brachial nerve

5-4. You find that many of your patients that have gone to the emergency department with chest pain have a negative set of initial cardiac enzymes. Most of those with a negative set of initial enzymes did not have a heart attack. You decide to evaluate 100 of your patients who have gone to the emergency department with chest pain to find out if an initial set of negative enzymes by itself is a good predictor of those that are not having a myocardial infarction (MI). Of those 100 patients, 20 of them had acute MIs. Of those 20, 10 had a positive set of enzymes initially. Of the 80 that did not have an acute MI, none of them had a positive set of initial enzymes. Given this information, what is the negative predictive value of the initial set of cardiac enzymes in your patient population?

a. 20%
b. 22%
c. 50%
d. 89%
e. 100%

5-5. A 20-month-old girl is admitted to a pediatric ward because she weighs only 15 lb. An extensive medical work-up does not reveal any organic cause for the child's failure to thrive. The child is listless and apathetic and does not smile. The parents rarely come to visit, and when they do, they do not pick the child up and do not play or interact with her. Which of the following statements best explains this scenario?

a. Lack of adequate emotional nurturance causes depression and failure to thrive in infants.
b. Neglected infants fail to thrive but do not have the intrapsychic structures necessary for experiencing depression.
c. Infants reared in institutions are likely to become autistic.
d. Neglected infants are at higher risk for developing schizophrenia.
e. Environmental variables have little impact on the health of infants as long as enough food is provided.

5-6. A 70-year-old nursing home resident was admitted to the hospital for pneumonia and treated for 10 days with levofloxacin. On discharge she was improved but developed diarrhea one week later. She had low-grade fever and mild abdominal pain with 2 to 3 watery, nonbloody stools per day. A cell culture cytotoxicity test for *Clostridium difficile*–associated disease was positive. The patient was treated with oral metronidazole, but did not improve, even after 10 days. Diarrhea has increased and fever and abdominal pain continue. What is the best next step in the management of this patient?

a. Obtain *C difficile* enzyme immunoassay.
b. Continue metronidazole for at least two more weeks.
c. Switch treatment to oral vancomycin.
d. Hospitalize patient for fulminant *C difficile*–associated disease.
e. Use synthetic fecal bacterial enema.

5-7. A 5-year-old boy presents with the severe rash shown in the photographs. The rash is pruritic, and it is especially intense in the flexural areas. The mother reports that the symptoms began in infancy (when it also involved the face) and that her 6-month-old child has similar symptoms. Which of the following is the most appropriate treatment of this condition?

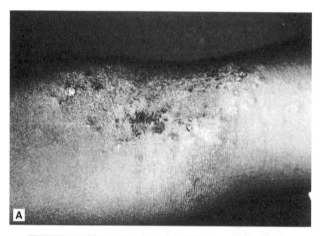

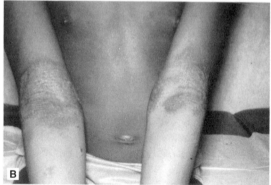

(Used with permission from Adelaide Hebert, MD.)

a. Coal-tar soaps and shampoo
b. Topical antifungal cream
c. Ultraviolet light therapy
d. Moisturizers and topical steroids
e. Topical antibiotics

5-8. You are evaluating an 18-year-old college student complaining of painful menstrual periods. She reports that she began menstruating at age 14. Since that time, her periods have always been associated with pain. The pain begins just prior to her period starting, and lasts for up to 3 days. She has associated nausea, fatigue, and headache. Her history and physical examination are normal, and you choose to treat her with a trial of oral contraceptives. Which of the following describes how oral contraceptives work to treat dysmenorrhea?

a. Suppression of prostaglandin synthesis
b. Suppression of prostaglandin release
c. Induction of endometrial hyperplasia
d. Increase in vasoconstriction of the uterus
e. Direct decrease of uterine resting tone

5-9. A 64-year-old man presents with acute exacerbation of chronic obstructive pulmonary disease. The patient had a long smoking history before quitting 2 years ago. In spite of his poor baseline lung function, he has been able to maintain an independent lifestyle. The patient is in obvious respiratory distress and appears tired. He has difficulty greeting you secondary to shortness of breath. Respiratory rate is 32/minute. Auscultation of the lungs reveals minimal air movement. ABGs show pH = 7.28, $Paco_2$ = 77, and Pao_2 = 54. One dose of IV methylprednisolone has already been administered. What is the best next step in the management of this patient's disease?

a. Urgent institution of BiPAP (bilevel positive airway pressure)
b. Urgent endotracheal intubation
c. Administration of 100% Fio_2 by face mask
d. Arrangement for admission to monitored ICU bed
e. IV levofloxacin

5-10. A 65-year-old man has an enterocutaneous fistula originating in the jejunum secondary to inflammatory bowel disease. Which of the following would be the most appropriate fluid for replacement of his enteric losses?

a. D5W
b. 3% normal saline
c. Ringer lactate solution
d. 0.9% sodium chloride
e. 6% sodium bicarbonate solution

5-11. A 41-year-old homosexual man is brought to medical attention by his partner because of headache, sluggish mentation, and impaired ambulation worsening over the previous week. The patient is known to be HIV seropositive, but has done well in the past and has not sought regular medical attention. On examination, his responses are slow and he has some difficulty sustaining attention. He has a right hemiparesis with increased reflexes on the right. Routine cell counts and chemistries are normal. A contrast head CT reveals several ring-enhancing lesions. Eventually, surgical aspiration of one of the lesions reveals that they are abscesses. Abscesses in the brain most often develop from which of the following?

a. Hematogenous spread of infection
b. Penetrating head wounds
c. Superinfection of neoplastic foci
d. Dental trauma
e. Neurosurgical intervention

5-12. An 82-year-old white female is admitted to the hospital for observation after presenting to the emergency department with dizziness. After being placed on a cardiac monitor in the ER, the rhythm strip below was recorded. There is no past history of cardiac disease, diabetes, or hypertension. With prompting, the patient discloses several prior episodes of transient dizziness and one episode of brief syncope in the past. Physical examination is unremarkable. Which of the following is the best plan of care?

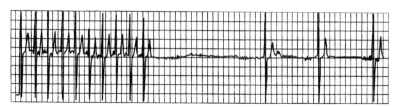

(Reproduced, with permission, from Kasper DL et al. Harrison's Principles of Internal Medicine, 15th ed. New York, NY: McGraw-Hill, 2001.)

a. Reassurance. This is a benign condition, and no direct therapy is needed.
b. Reassurance. The patient may not drive until she is symptom free, but otherwise no direct therapy is needed.
c. Nuclear cardiac stress testing; treatment depending on results.
d. Begin therapy with aspirin.
e. Arrange placement of a permanent pacemaker.

5-13. A 16-year-old camp counselor sees you to evaluate a severely pruritic rash. You note pruritic erythematous papules in between his fingers, on his wrists, and around his waist. For which of the following is this distribution characteristic?

a. Flea bites
b. Bedbugs
c. Body lice
d. Scabies
e. Chigger bites

5-14. Three policemen, with difficulty, drag an agitated and very combative young man into an emergency room. Once there, he is restrained because he reacts with rage and tries to hit anyone who approaches him. When it is finally safe to approach him, the resident on call notices that the patient has very prominent vertical nystagmus. Shortly thereafter, the patient has a generalized seizure. Which of the following substances of abuse is most likely to produce this presentation?

a. Amphetamine
b. PCP
c. Cocaine
d. Meperidine
e. LSD

5-15. A 49-year-old man presents to the ED with nausea, vomiting, and abdominal pain that began approximately 2 days ago. The patient states that he usually drinks a six-pack of beer daily, but increased his drinking to two six-packs daily over the last week because of pressures at work. He notes decreased appetite over the last 3 days and states he has not had anything to eat in 2 days. His BP is 125/75 mm Hg, HR is 105 beats per minute, and RR is 20 breaths per minute. You note generalized abdominal tenderness on examination. Laboratory results reveal the following:

White blood cells (WBC) 9000/μL
Hematocrit 48%
Platelets 210/μL
Aspartate transaminase (AST) 85 U/L
Alanine transaminase (ALT) 60 U/L

Alkaline phosphatase 75 U/L
Total bilirubin 0.5 mg/dL
Lipase 40 IU

Sodium 131 mEq/L
Potassium 3.5 mEq/L
Chloride 101 mEq/L
Bicarbonate 10 mEq/L
Blood urea nitrogen (BUN)
  9 mg/dL
Creatinine 0.5 mg/dL
Glucose 190 mg/dL
Nitroprusside test weakly
  positive for ketones

Which of the following is the mainstay of therapy for patients with this condition?

a. Normal saline (NS) solution
b. Half normal saline ($^1/_2$ NS)
c. Glucose solution (D_5W)
d. Solution containing both saline and glucose (D_5/NS or D_5 $^1/_2$ NS)
e. The type of solution is irrelevant

5-16. A 21-year-old woman presents to the emergency room in active labor. She has had no prenatal care, but her last menstrual period was approximately 9 months prior. Her membranes are artificially ruptured, yielding no amniotic fluid. She delivers an 1800-g (4-lb) term infant who develops significant respiratory distress immediately at birth. The first chest radiograph on this infant demonstrates hypoplastic lungs. After this infant is stabilized, which of the following is the most appropriate next step for this infant?

a. Cardiac catheterization
b. Renal ultrasound
c. MRI of the brain
d. Liver and spleen scan
e. Upper GI

5-17. A 50-year-old female is 5 ft 7 in tall and weighs 185 lb. There is a family history of diabetes mellitus. Fasting blood glucose (FBG) is 160 mg/dL and 155 mg/dL on two occasions. HgA1c is 7.8%. You educate the patient on medical nutrition therapy. She returns for reevaluation in 8 weeks. She states she has followed diet and exercise recommendations but her FBG remains between 130 and 140 and HgA1C is 7.3%. She is asymptomatic, and physical examination shows no abnormalities. Which of the following is the treatment of choice?

a. Thiazolidinediones
b. Encourage compliance with medical nutrition therapy
c. Insulin
d. Metformin
e. Observation with repeat HgA1C in 6 weeks.

5-18. A 25-year-old G3P2 at 39 weeks is admitted in labor at 5 cm dilated. The fetal heart rate tracing is reactive. Two hours later, she is reexamined and her cervix is unchanged at 5 cm dilated. An IUPC is placed and the patient is noted to have 280 Montevideo units (MUV) by the IUPC. After an additional 2 hours of labor, the patient is noted to still be 5 cm dilated. The fetal heart rate tracing remains reactive. Which of the following is the best next step in the management of this labor?

a. Perform a cesarean section
b. Continue to wait and observe the patient
c. Augment labor with Pitocin
d. Attempt delivery via vacuum extraction
e. Perform an operative delivery with forceps

5-19. The mother of one of your regular patients calls your office. She reports that her daughter has a 3-day history of subjective fever, hoarseness, and a bad barking cough. You arrange for her to be seen in your office that morning. Upon seeing this child, you would expect to find which of the following?

a. A temperature greater than 38.9°C (102°F)
b. Expiratory stridor
c. Infection with parainfluenza virus
d. Hyperinflation on chest x-ray
e. A child between 6 and 8 years of age

5-20. You are evaluating a 25-year-old woman who reports frequent UTIs since getting married last year. In the last 12 months, she has had five documented infections that have responded well to antibiotic therapy. She has tried voiding after intercourse, she discontinued her use of a diaphragm, and tried acidification of her urine using oral ascorbic acid, but none of those measures decreased the incidence of infections. At this point, which of the following would be an acceptable prophylactic measure?

a. An antibiotic prescription for the usual 3-day regimen with refills, to be used when symptoms occur
b. Single dose antibiotic therapy once daily at bedtime for 12 months
c. Single dose antibiotic therapy once daily at bedtime for 2 years
d. Single dose antibiotic therapy after sexual intercourse
e. Antibiotics for 3 days after sexual intercourse

5-21. A 30-year-old quadriplegic male presents to the emergency room with fever, dyspnea, and a cough. He has a chronic indwelling Foley catheter. Recurrent urinary tract infections have been a problem for a number of years. He has been on therapy to suppress the urinary tract infections. On examination, mild wheezing is audible over both lungs. A diffuse erythematous rash is noted. The chest x-ray shows a diffuse alveolar infiltrate. The CBC reveals a WBC of 13,500, with 50% segmented cells, 30% lymphocytes, and 20% eosinophils. Which of the following is the most likely diagnosis?

a. Sepsis with ARDS secondary to urinary tract infection
b. Healthcare-related pneumonia
c. A drug reaction to one of his medications
d. An acute exacerbation of COPD
e. Lymphocytic interstitial pneumonitis

5-22. A 49-year-old man was the restrained driver in a motor vehicle collision. He decelerated rapidly in order to avoid hitting another car and swerved into a ditch. He complains of chest pain. Which of the following findings on chest x-ray would be most suspicious for an aortic injury?

a. Multiple right-sided rib fractures
b. A left pulmonary contusion
c. A left pneumothorax
d. Widening of the mediastinum greater than 8 cm
e. Pneumomediastinum

Questions 23 to 28

Choose the toxin that is most likely to produce each clinical scenario. Each lettered option may be used once, more than once, or not at all.

a. Lead
b. Arsenic
c. Manganese
d. Mercury
e. Carbon monoxide
f. Ergot
g. Nitrous oxide

5-23. A man working in a poorly regulated felt-processing plant develops tremors and memory disturbances over the course of months. He seeks medical help when tremors of his tongue and lips became embarrassing and he is injured during a fall. His family notes progressive irritability and depression. On neurologic examination, he has prominent gait ataxia, limb and facial tremors, and decreased pain and temperature sense in his feet.

5-24. While vacationing in Latin America, a student buys a brightly painted glazed ceramic pitcher. He drinks orange juice from the pitcher every night while studying. Within 4 months of starting this practice, he develops weakness in both wrists. He consults a physician, who finds weakness on dorsiflexion of both hands, unassociated with any sensory deficits. An EMG reveals evidence of a peripheral motor neuropathy.

5-25. A 45-year-old woman reports to the police her discovery that her husband has added a suspicious material to her food. She has experienced matrimonial problems for several years and has developed progressive fatigue with frequent headache over the prior 3 months. She consulted a physician when she developed recurrent bouts of severe stomach pain and was told by neighbors that she had been talking to herself and attacking invisible assailants. The physician noted that she had an unexplained anemia and white lines running transversely across her fingernails. She also has had problems with her memory, excessive drowsiness, and a sensorimotor neuropathy with absent tendon reflexes. The physician sent a sample of her hair for analysis and found a neurotoxin present.

5-26. An Eastern European immigrant who recently arrived in the United States is brought to the emergency room after a seizure. He first developed seizures at the age of 30 and never received treatment. Neurologic examination reveals fasciculations and occasional myoclonus. He is ataxic and has absent deep tendon reflexes. A sensory neuropathy is evident in his legs. Ulcers are evident on his fingers and toes. He acknowledges that his diet was very limited before he immigrated to the United States, and states that most of his calories were derived from rye grains.

5-27. A 38-year-old miner develops a shuffling gait, tremor, and drooling. His speech is difficult to understand and trails off in volume until it is inaudible. He consults a physician because of easy fatigability and frequent falls. Cogwheel rigidity is evident in his arms and legs. His tremor is most evident when his limbs are at rest.

5-28. A 35-year-old woman is rescued from a burning building. She is comatose on arrival in the ER. Her skin is cyanotic. Computed tomography (CT) scan of her head shows mild cerebral edema. After intensive care in a burn unit, she recovers markedly, but 2 weeks later, she begins to develop dystonic posturing and bradykinesia. A CT scan now shows hypodensities in the globus pallidum bilaterally.

5-29. A 25-year-old man presents to the ED complaining of dull periumbilical pain that migrated to his RLQ over the last hour. He states that he has no appetite and vomited twice. His BP is 125/75 mm Hg, HR is 87 beats per minute, temperature is 100.6°F, and RR is 16 breaths per minute. Laboratory results reveal WBC 11,000/µL, hematocrit 48%, platelets 170/µL. On physical examination, the patient complains of pain when you flex his knee with internal rotation at his hip. What is the name of this sign?

a. Obturator
b. Psoas
c. Rovsing
d. McBurney
e. Murphy

5-30. You are evaluating a 41-year-old man with the acute onset of low back pain. It started 2 days ago while he was putting his child into his car seat. The pain radiates to his right leg. On examination, his range of motion is limited but his neurological examination is normal. When you lay him on his back and raise his fully extended leg about 30° by the heel, he reports pain below the knee. Which of the following is the most likely diagnosis?

a.   Back strain
b.   An inflammatory condition
c.   Disk herniation
d.   Compression fracture
e.   Neoplasm

5-31. A 15-year-old woman presents to your office for her first well-woman examination while she is on summer break from school. She denies any medical problems or prior surgeries. She had chicken pox at age 4. Her menses started at the age of 12 and are regular. She has recently become sexually active with her 16-year-old boyfriend. She states that they use condoms for contraception. Her physical examination is normal. Which of the following vaccines is appropriate to administer to this patient?

a.   Hepatitis A vaccine
b.   Pneumococcal vaccine
c.   Varicella vaccine
d.   Hepatitis B vaccine
e.   Influenza vaccine

5-32. A 38-year-old female presents to your office with complaints of fatigue and generalized weakness for 6 weeks. She experiences stiffness in her hands and wrists for an hour after waking, and has taken nonsteroidal anti-inflammatory medication with some relief. Two weeks ago, she noticed that her knuckles were red and tender. Her past medical history is unremarkable, and she takes no medications. On examination, her temperature is 100°F. Erythema with edema is present at most MCP joints. She has minimally decreased muscle strength. Her labs include

WBC: 12,000
Hemoglobin: 10.6 g/dL
Rheumatoid factor: negative
Antibodies to citrulline-containing proteins (anti-CCP): positive
ESR: 62
Hand x-ray: juxtaarticular osteopenia of the MCP joints

Scheduled nonsteroidal anti-inflammatories are started with appropriate monitoring. After one month her pain is unchanged. What is the most appropriate next step in her treatment?

a. Physical therapy.
b. Referral to a rheumatologist.
c. Begin IV TNF monoclonal antibodies.
d. Begin allopurinol.
e. Begin doxycycline 100mg twice daily for 30 days.

5-33. You are admitting to the hospital a 3-month-old infant who has been having poor feeding, emesis, and diarrhea for 3 days. In the emergency center, her electrolytes were found to be: sodium 157 mEq/L, potassium 2.6 mEq/L, chloride 120 mEq/L, bicarbonate 14 mEq/L, creatinine 1.8 mEq/L, blood urea nitrogen (BUN) 68 mEq/L, and glucose 195 mEq/L. She was given a fluid bolus in the emergency center and has subsequently produced urine. Which of the following is the most appropriate next step in her management?

a. Slow rehydration over 48 hours
b. Continued rapid volume expansion with $^{1}/_{4}$ normal saline
c. Packed red blood cells (RBCs)
d. Rehydration with free water
e. Urinary electrolytes

5-34. Parents bring a 5-day-old infant to your office. The mother is O negative and was Coombs positive at delivery. The term child weighed 3055 g (6 lb, 1 oz) at birth and had measured baseline hemoglobin of 16 g/dL and a total serum bilirubin of 3 mg/dL. He passed a black tarlike stool within the first 24 hours of life. He was discharged at 30 hours of life with a stable axillary temperature of 36.5°C (97.7°F). Today the infant's weight is 3000 g, his axillary temperature is 35°C (95°F), and he is jaundiced to the chest. Parents report frequent yellow, seedy stool. You redraw labs and find his hemoglobin is now 14 g/dL, and his total serum bilirubin is 13 mg/dL. The change in which of the following parameters is of most concern?

a. Hemoglobin
b. Temperature
c. Body weight
d. Bilirubin
e. Stool

5-35. A 42-year-old man with no history of use of NSAIDs presents with recurrent gastritis. Infection with *Helicobacter pylori* is suspected. Which of the following is most accurate?

a. Morphologically, the bacteria are a gram-positive, tennis-racket–shaped organism.
b. Diagnosis can be made by serologic testing or urea breath tests.
c. Diagnosis is most routinely achieved via culturing endoscopic scrapings.
d. The most effective way to treat and prevent recurrence of this patient's gastritis is through the use of single-drug therapy aimed at eradicating *H pylori*.
e. The organism is easily eradicated.

5-36. A 22-year-old college student notices a bulge in his right groin. It is accentuated with coughing, but is easily reducible. Which of the following hernias follows the path of the spermatic cord within the cremaster muscle?

a. Femoral
b. Direct inguinal
c. Indirect inguinal
d. Spigelian
e. Interparietal

5-37. Which of the following serum level ranges is the target for lithium use in acute mania?

a. 0.5 to 1.0 meq/L
b. 1.0 to 1.5 meq/L
c. 1.5 to 2.0 meq/L
d. 2.0 to 2.5 meq/L
e. 2.5 to 3.0 meq/L

Questions 38 to 40

Match the clinical presentation with the likely cause of the patient's renal failure. Each lettered option may be used once, more than once, or not at all.

a. Prerenal azotemia because of intravascular volume depletion
b. Ischemia-induced acute tubular necrosis
c. Nephrotoxin-induced acute tubular necrosis
d. Acute interstitial nephritis
e. Postrenal azotemia because of obstructive uropathy
f. Postinfectious glomerulonephritis
g. Acute cortical necrosis

5-38. A patient is admitted to the hospital with a nursing-home acquired pneumonia. His blood pressure is normal and the extremities well-perfused. Admission creatinine is 1.2 mg/dL. UA is clear. The patient is treated on the floor with piperacillin/tazobactam and improves clinically. On the fourth hospital day, the patient notes a nonpruritic rash over the abdomen. The creatinine has risen to 2.2 mg/dL. The urinalysis shows 2+ protein, 10 to 15 WBC/HPF, and no casts or RBCs.

5-39. A 62-year-old man is admitted with pneumonia and severe sepsis. Vasopressors are required to maintain peripheral perfusion, and mechanical ventilation is needed because of ARDS. Admission creatinine is 1.0 mg/dL but rises by the second hospital day to 2.2 mg/dL. Urine output is 300 cc/24 hours. UA shows renal tubular epithelial cells and some muddy brown casts. The fractional excretion of sodium is 3.45.

5-40. A 76-year-old man is admitted with pneumonia. He has a history of diabetes mellitus. Admission creatinine is 1.2 mg/dL. He responds to ceftriaxone and azithromycin. He develops occasional urinary incontinence treated with anticholinergics, but his overall status improves and he is ready for discharge by the fifth hospital day. On that morning, however, he develops urinary hesitancy and slight suprapubic tenderness. The creatinine is found to be 3.0 mg/dL; UA is clear with no RBCs, WBCs or protein.

5-41. A 21-year-old woman presents to the ED complaining of lightheadedness. Her symptoms appeared 45 minutes ago. She has no other symptoms and is not on any medications. She has a medical history of mitral valve prolapse. Her HR is 170 beats per minute and BP is 105/55 mm Hg. Physical examination is unremarkable. After administering the appropriate medication, her HR slows down and her symptoms resolve. You repeat a 12-lead ECG that shows a rate of 89 beats per minute with a regular rhythm. The PR interval measures 100 msec and there is a slurred upstroke of the QRS complex. Based on this information, which of the following is the most likely diagnosis?

a. Ventricular tachycardia
b. Atrial flutter with 3:1 block
c. Atrial fibrillation
d. Lown-Ganong-Levine (LGL) syndrome
f. Wolff-Parkinson-White (WPW) syndrome

5-42. A 90-year-old G5P5 with multiple medical problems is brought into your gynecology clinic accompanied by her granddaughter. The patient has hypertension, chronic anemia, coronary artery disease, and osteoporosis. She is mentally alert and oriented and lives in an assisted living facility. She takes numerous medications, but is very functional at the current time. She is a widow and not sexually active. Her chief complaint is a sensation of heaviness and pressure in the vagina. She denies any significant urinary or bowel problems. On performance of a physical examination, you note that the cervix is just inside the level of the introitus. Based on the physical examination, which of the following is the most likely diagnosis?

a. Normal examination
b. First-degree uterine prolapse
c. Second-degree uterine prolapse
d. Third-degree uterine prolapse
e. Complete procidentia

Questions 43 to 44

5-43. A 34-year-old woman comes to the physician with the chief complaint of abdominal pain. She states that she has been reading on the internet and is convinced that she has ovarian cancer. She says that she is particularly concerned because the other physicians she has seen for this pain have all told her that she does not have cancer, and she has been having the pain for over 8 months. She reports that she has undergone pelvic examinations, ultrasounds, and other diagnostic work-ups, all of which have been negative. She tells the physician that she is initially reassured by the negative tests, but then the pain returns and she becomes convinced that she has cancer again. She notes that she has taken so much time off from work in the past 8 months that she has been reprimanded by her boss. Which of the following is the most likely diagnosis?

a. Pain disorder
b. Malingering
c. Factitious disorder
d. Hypochondriasis
e. Conversion disorder

5-44. Which of the following courses of action is most likely to be helpful in the case of the woman in the vignette above?

a. Refer the patient to psychotherapy
b. Start the patient on an antidepressant
c. Have the patient see a primary care physician at regular intervals
d. Begin a diagnostic work-up for ovarian cancer
e. Start the patient on an antipsychotic for her delusional belief

5-45. A 30-year-old man is brought to the ED by emergency medical service (EMS) in respiratory distress. His initial vitals include a HR of 109 beats per minute, a BP of 180/90 mm Hg, and an RR of 20 breaths per minute with an oxygen saturation of 92% on room air. A chest x-ray shows a bilateral diffuse infiltrative process. A subsequent toxicologic screen is positive. Which of the following agents is most likely responsible for this patient's presentation?

a. Cannabis
b. Opioid
c. Crack cocaine
d. Methamphetamine
e. Ethanol

5-46. A 62-year-old man has been diagnosed with an abdominal aortic aneurysm. He is told that he is at high risk for aneurysm rupture, which would almost certainly kill him. Although a surgical procedure could dramatically reduce this risk, the operation itself has risks, including postoperative paraplegia. The arteria radicularis magna (artery of Adamkiewicz) enters at approximately what level?

a. C2 to C5
b. C5 to C8
c. T2 to T8
d. T10 to L1
e. L4 to S4

Block 6

Questions

6-1. You are discussing cancer screening with a patient. Her father was diagnosed with colorectal cancer at age 58. When should you recommend she begins colorectal cancer screening?

a. 40 years
b. 48 years
c. 50 years
d. 58 years
e. 60 years

6-2. A 32-year-old man develops weakness in his hands over the course of 3 months. Further questioning reveals that he is also having trouble with swallowing. He occasionally slurs his words and has noticed progressive weakness in his cough over the preceding 4 weeks. The weakness is not substantially worse later in the day. He has no sensory symptoms associated with his weakness. Sexual function, bladder and bowel control, hearing, vision, and balance are all alleged to be unchanged. The examining physician discovers marked atrophy of the interosseous muscles of both hands. Deep tendon reflexes are hyperactive in the arms and the legs. Extensor plantar responses are present bilaterally. Rectal sphincter tone is normal. This patient's illness characteristically produces electromyographic changes that include which of the following?

a. Fibrillations
b. Markedly slowed nerve conduction velocities
c. Impaired sensory nerve action potentials
d. H reflexes
e. No abnormalities

6-3. The 1-year-old boy in the photograph below, who recently had a circumcision, requires an additional operation on his genitalia that will probably eliminate his risk of which of the following?

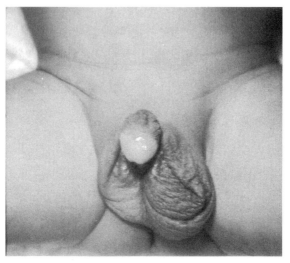

(Used with permission from Michael L. Ritchey, MD.)

a. Testicular malignancy
b. Decreased sperm count
c. Torsion of testes
d. Urinary tract infection
e. Epididymitis

6-4. A mother notices an abdominal mass in her 3-year-old son while giving him a bath. There is no history of any symptoms, but the boy's blood pressure is elevated at 105/85 mm Hg. Metastatic workup is negative and the patient is explored. The mass shown here is found within the left kidney. Which of the following statements best describes this disease?

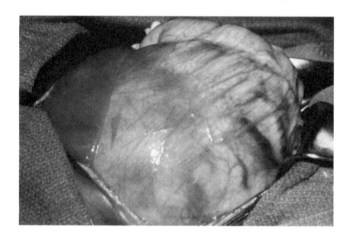

a. This tumor is associated with aniridia, hemihypertrophy, and cryptorchidism.
b. The majority of patients present with an asymptomatic abdominal mass and hematuria.
c. Treatment with surgical excision, radiation, and chemotherapy results in survival of less than 60% even in histologically low-grade tumors.
d. Surgical excision is curative and no further treatment is ordinarily advised.
e. This tumor is the most common abdominal malignancy of childhood.

6-5. A 26-year-old woman presents to the ED with an acute onset of dyspnea after falling down a few steps. The patient denies any loss of consciousness and reports feeling short of breath. Her initial chest x-ray appears normal; however she continues to be symptomatic with stable vital signs. Which of the following procedures should be performed next?

a. Repeat upright chest x-ray
b. Inspiratory and expiratory chest radiographs
c. Chest CT scan
d. Chest thoracostomy
e. Chest thoracotomy

6-6. A mentally retarded male adolescent who has been increasingly aggressive and agitated receives several consecutive IM doses of haloperidol, totaling 30 mg in 24 hours, as a chemical restraint. The next day, he is rigid, confused, and unresponsive. His blood pressure is 150/95 mm Hg, his pulse is 110 beats/min, and his temperature is 38.9°C (102°F). Both his WBC count and CPK levels are very high. Which of the following is the most likely diagnosis?

a. Acute dystonic reaction
b. Neuroleptic-induced Parkinson disease
c. Malignant hyperthermia
d. Neuroleptic malignant syndrome
e. Catatonia

6-7. A 32-year-old male presents to your office with concern about progressive fatigue and lower extremity edema. He has experienced decreased exercise tolerance over the past few months, and occasionally awakens coughing at night. Past medical history is significant for sickle cell anemia and diabetes mellitus. He has had multiple admissions to the hospital secondary to vaso-occlusive crises since the age of three. Physical examination reveals a displaced PMI, but is otherwise unremarkable. ECG shows a first degree AV block and low voltage. Chest x-ray shows an enlarged cardiac silhouette with clear lung fields. Which of the following would be the best initial diagnostic approach?

a. Order serum iron, iron-binding capacity, and ferritin level.
b. Order brain-natriuretic peptide (BNP)
c. Order CT scan of the chest.
d. Arrange for placement of a 24-hour ambulatory cardiac monitor.
e. Arrange for cardiac catheterization.

6-8. Physical examination of a patient who has had a spinal cord infarct reveals preservation of some sensation in the feet. Which of the following would be the most intact modality?

a. Joint proprioception
b. Pain
c. Temperature
d. Two-point discrimination
e. Graphesthesia

Questions 9 to 10

6-9. A 43-year-old woman comes to the emergency room with a temperature of 38.3°C (101°F) and a large suppurating ulcer on her left shoulder. This is the third such episode for this woman. Her physical examination is otherwise normal, except for the presence of multiple scars on her abdomen. Which of the following is the most likely diagnosis?

a. Malingering
b. Somatoform disorder
c. Borderline personality disorder
d. Factitious disorder
e. Body dysmorphic disorder

6-10. Which of the following etiologies is most likely underlying the behavior of the woman in the vignette above?

a. Primary gain
b. Secondary gain
c. Psychosis
d. Marginal intellectual function
e. Drug-seeking behavior

6-11. A patient presents to your office in distress without an appointment. He is 23 years old and is complaining of severe chest pain. He reports a family history of coronary disease, complains of frequent "heartburn," and says he is recovering from a recent viral upper respiratory infection. He smokes one pack of cigarettes a day, and admits to illegal drug use in the past. On examination, his blood pressure is 138/90 mm Hg, his pulse is 126 beats per minute and regular, and he is diaphoretic. His examination is otherwise unremarkable. His electrocardiogram (ECG) shows myocardial ischemia. Which of his historical features are most suggestive that myocardial ischemia would be the cause of his symptoms?

a. Family history of coronary disease
b. History of "heartburn"
c. Recent viral upper respiratory infection
d. Smoking history
e. Drug use

6-12. A 9-year-old girl is playing in a wooded area of her backyard. She notices a furry animal in the brush. As it does not seem to fear her, she approaches to pet it. As soon as she touches the creature, it bites her and runs away. Her parents bring her to the emergency room for evaluation. The emergency room physician is extremely concerned that the patient may have been exposed to a deadly virus and orders immediate injections of immunoglobulin. From the brain, this pathogen establishes itself for transmission to another host by spreading to which of the following?

a. Intestines
b. Nasopharynx
c. Lungs
d. Bladder
e. Salivary glands

6-13. The parents of a previously healthy 2-year-old child note her to be pale and bring her to your clinic for evaluation. She currently has no fever, nausea, emesis, bone pain, or other complaints. Her examination is significant for pallor, tachycardia, and a systolic ejection murmur, but she has no organomegaly. Her complete blood count (CBC) reveals a hemoglobin of 4 g/dL, normal indices for age, a WBC count of 6.5/µL, and a platelet count of 750,000/µL. Her reticulocyte count is 0%. Coombs test is negative. Her peripheral blood smear shows no blast forms and no fragments. Red blood cell (RBC) adenosine deaminase levels are normal. A bone marrow reveals markedly decreased erythroid precursors. Which of the following is this child's likely diagnosis?

a. Diamond-Blackfan anemia
b. Sickle-cell anemia
c. Pearson marrow-pancreas syndrome
d. Iron deficiency anemia
e. Transient erythroblastopenia of childhood

6-14. A 55-year-old man presents to the ED at 2:00 AM with left-sided chest pain that radiates down his left arm. He takes a β-blocker for hypertension, a proton-pump inhibitor for gastroesophageal reflux disease, and an antilipid agent for high cholesterol. He also took sildenafil the previous night for erectile dysfunction. His BP is 130/70 mm Hg and HR is 77 beats per minute. Which of the following medication is contraindicated in this patient?

a. Aspirin
b. Unfractionated heparin
c. Nitroglycerin
d. Metoprolol
e. Morphine sulfate

6-15. You are caring for a 35-year-old woman in the hospital, admitted for cellulitis. She also has a long history of migraine headaches. On day 2 of her hospitalization, she becomes diaphoretic, restless, and irritable. Within hours, she is complaining of severe pain, abdominal cramps, and diarrhea. Which of the following would most likely be present in her urine toxicology screen?

a. Cocaine
b. Marijuana
c. Opiates
d. 3,4-Methylenedioxymethampheatmine (MDMA or ecstasy)
e. Benzodiazepines

6-16. A healthy 23-year-old G1P0 has had an uncomplicated pregnancy to date. She is disappointed because she is 40 weeks gestational age by good dates and a first-trimester ultrasound. She feels like she has been pregnant forever, and wants to have her baby now. The patient reports good fetal movement; she has been doing kick counts for the past several days and reports that the baby moves about eight times an hour on average. On physical examination, her cervix is firm, posterior, 50% effaced, and 1 cm dilated, and the vertex is at a-1 station. As her obstetrician, which of the following should you recommend to the patient?

a. She should be admitted for an immediate cesarean section.
b. She should be admitted for Pitocin induction.
c. You will schedule a cesarean section in 1 week if she has not undergone spontaneous labor in the meantime.
d. She should continue to monitor kick counts and to return to your office in 1 week to reassess the situation.

6-17. A 39-year-old previously healthy male is hospitalized for 2 weeks with epigastric pain radiating to his back, nausea, and vomiting. Initial laboratory values revealed an elevated amylase level consistent with acute pancreatitis. Five weeks following discharge, he complains of early satiety, epigastric pain, and fevers. On presentation, his temperature is 38.9°C (102°F) and his heart rate is 120 beats per minute; his white blood cell (WBC) count is 24,000/mm³ and his amylase level is normal. He undergoes a CT scan demonstrating a 6-cm by 6-cm rim-enhancing fluid collection in the body of the pancreas. Which of the following would be the most definitive management of the fluid collection?

a. Antibiotic therapy alone
b. CT-guided aspiration with repeat imaging in 2 to 3 days
c. Antibiotics and CT-guided aspiration with repeat imaging in 2 to 3 days
d. Antibiotics and percutaneous catheter drainage
e. Surgical internal drainage of the fluid collection with a cyst-gastrostomy or Roux-en-Y cyst-jejunostomy

Questions 18 to 20

Match each symptom or sign with the appropriate disease. Each lettered option may be used once, more than once, or not at all.

a. Subacute thyroiditis
b. Graves disease
c. Factitious hyperthyroidism
d. Struma ovarii
e. Multinodular goiter
f. Thyroid nodule
g. Iodide deficiency
h. TSH-secreting pituitary adenoma

6-18. 20-year-old female presents with tachycardia, tremor, and heat intolerance. On physical examination, no thyromegaly is noted, but she does have RLQ fullness on pelvic examination. TSH is < 0.01, and radionuclide scan reveals low uptake in the thyroid gland.

6-19. A male nursing assistant presents with weakness and tremor. Examination shows no ophthalmopathy or pretibial myxedema. No thyroid tissue is palpable. T_4 is elevated; radioactive iodine uptake is reduced.

6-20. A 20-year-old presents after recent upper respiratory infection. She complains of neck pain and heat intolerance. The thyroid is tender. Erythrocyte sedimentation rate is elevated; free thyroxine value is modestly elevated.

6-21. A 23-year-old woman is brought to the emergency room from a halfway house, where she apparently swallowed a handful of pills. The patient complains of shortness of breath and tinnitus, but refuses to identify the pills she ingested. Pertinent laboratory values are as follows:

Arterial blood gases: pH 7.45, P_{CO_2} 12 mm Hg, P_{O_2} 126 mm Hg.
Serum electrolytes (mEq/L): Na^+ 138, K^+ 4.8, Cl^- 102, HCO_3^- 8.

An overdose of which of the following drugs would be most likely to cause the acid–base disturbance in this patient?

a. Phenformin
b. Aspirin
c. Barbiturates
d. Methanol
e. Diazepam (Valium)

6-22. A 38-year-old HIV-positive man follows up in your office for routine care. Unfortunately, his antiretroviral therapy is failing, and his CD4 count is falling. At his last two visits, his CD4 count has been less than 65 lymphocytes/mm^3. Prophylaxis for which of the following should be instituted at this time?

a. *Mycobacterium avium* complex
b. Fungal infections
c. Herpes simplex
d. Herpes zoster
e. Cytomegalovirus

6-23. A 45-year-old housewife has been drinking in secret for several years. She started with one or two small glasses of Irish cream per night to help her sleep, but, over time, her nightly intake has increased to four to five shots of hard liquor. Now she needs a few glasses of wine in the early afternoon to prevent shakiness and anxiety. During the past year, she could not take part in several important family events, including her son's high school graduation, because she was too ill or she did not want to risk missing her nightly drinking. She is ashamed of her secret and has tried to limit her alcohol intake but without success. Which of the following is the most likely diagnosis?

a. Alcohol abuse
b. Alcohol addiction
c. Addictive personality disorder
d. Alcohol dependence
e. Alcohol-induced mood disorder

6-24. A newborn child is being examined. During ophthalmologic evaluation, it is noticed that the red reflex is absent. Which of the following could this indicate?

a. Congenital cataracts
b. Chorioretinitis
c. Retinitis pigmentosa
d. Optic atrophy
e. Holoprosencephaly

6-25. A 15-year-old boy has been immobilized in a double hip spica cast for 6 weeks after having fractured his femur in a skiing accident. He has become depressed and listless during the past few days and has complained of nausea and constipation. He is found to have microscopic hematuria and a blood pressure of 150/100 mm Hg. Which of the following is the most appropriate course of action?

a. Request a psychiatric evaluation
b. Check blood pressure every 2 hours for 2 days
c. Collect urine for measurement of the calcium to creatinine ratio
d. Order a renal sonogram and intravenous pyelogram (IVP)
e. Measure 24-hour urinary protein

6-26. A 28-year-old woman comes to you for wart removal. On examination, she has a single wart on the lateral aspect of her index finger near the distal interphalangeal joint. She has no other medical conditions, but is trying to become pregnant. Her last period was 4 weeks ago. Which of the following treatment options would be best in this situation?

a. Topical treatment with liquid nitrogen
b. Topical treatment with podophyllum resin
c. Topical treatment with local interferon inducer like Imiquimod
d. CO_2 laser treatment
e. Injection with bleomycin

6-27. A 59-year-old man presents to the ED complaining of vomiting and sharp abdominal pain in the epigastric area that began abruptly this afternoon. He describes feeling nauseated and has no appetite. Laboratory results reveal WBC 18,000/μL, hematocrit 48%, platelets 110/μL, AST 275 U/L, ALT 125 U/L, alkaline phosphatase 75 U/L, amylase 1150 U/L, lipase 1450 IU, LDH 400 U/L, sodium 135 mEq/L, potassium 3.5 mEq/L, chloride 110 mEq/L, bicarbonate 20 mEq/L, BUN 20 mg/dL, creatinine 1.5 mg/dL, and glucose 250 mg/dL. Which of the following laboratory results correlate with the poorest prognosis?

a. Amylase 950, lipase 1250, LDH 400
b. Lipase 1250, LDH 400, bicarbonate 20
c. Lipase 1250, creatinine 1.5, potassium 3.5
d. WBC 18,000, LDH 400, glucose 250
e. WBC 18,000, amylase 950, lipase 1250

6-28. An 84-year-old woman develops confusion and agitation after surgery for hip fracture. Her family reports that prior to her hospitalization she functioned independently at home, although requiring help with balancing her checkbook and paying bills. Her current medications include intravenous fentanyl for pain control, lorazepam for control of her agitation, and DVT prophylaxis. She has also been started on ciprofloxacin for pyuria (culture pending). In addition to frequent reorientation of the patient, which of the following series of actions would best manage this patient's delirium?

a. Increase lorazepam to more effective dose, repeat urinalysis.
b. Discontinue lorazepam, remove Foley catheter, add haloperidol for severe agitation, and change to nonfluoroquinolone antibiotic.
c. Continue lorazepam at current dose, discontinue fentanyl, add soft restraints.
d. Continue lorazepam at current dose, add alprazolam 0.25 mg for severe agitation, repeat urinalysis, restrain patient to prevent self harm.
e. Discontinue lorazepam, remove Foley catheter, add alprazolam 0.25 mg for severe agitation, place the patient on telemetry.

6-29. A 3-year-old girl is admitted with the x-ray shown below. The child lives with her parents and a 6-week-old brother. Her grandfather stayed with the family for 2 months before his return to the West Indies 1 month ago. The grandfather had a 3-month history of weight loss, fever, and hemoptysis. Appropriate management of this problem includes which of the following?

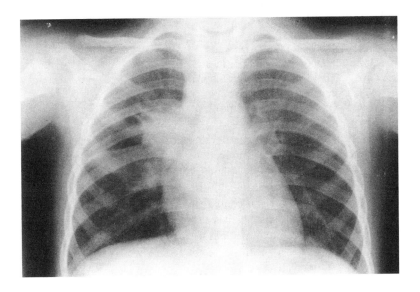

a. Bronchoscopy and culture of washings for all family members
b. Placement of a Mantoux test on the 6-week-old sibling
c. Isolating the 3-year-old patient for 1 month
d. Treating the 3-year-old patient with isoniazid (INH) and rifampin
e. HIV testing for all family members

Questions 30 to 31

6-30. A 61-year-old, right-handed man presents with involuntary twitches of his left hand. He first noticed between 6 months and 1 year ago that when he is at rest, his left hand shakes. He can stop the shaking by looking at his hand and concentrating. The shaking does not impair his activities in any way. He has no trouble holding a glass of water. There is no tremor in his right hand, and his lower extremities are not affected. He has had no trouble walking, and there have been no falls. There have been no behavioral or language changes. On examination, a tremor of the left hand is evident when the man is distracted. His handwriting is mildly tremulous. He has bilateral cogwheel rigidity with contralateral activation, which is worse on the left. His rapid alternating movements are bradykinetic on the left. Which of the following neurological structures is most likely dysfunctional?

a. Cerebral cortex
b. Peripheral nerves
c. Cerebral white matter
d. Brainstem nuclei
e. Cerebellum

6-31. The patient above becomes physically violent in the emergency room, attempting to strike a nurse and struggling with security. Which of the following actions should the psychiatrist take now?

a. Order full leather restraints.
b. Admit the patient to the inpatient psychiatry unit.
c. Offer the patient 5 mg of haloperidol PO.
d. Attempt to find out why the patient is so upset.
e. Assist security in restraining the patient.

6-32. A 62-year-old woman undergoes a lysis of adhesions and bowel resection for small-bowel obstruction secondary to radiation enteritis after treatment for ovarian cancer. A jejunostomy is placed to facilitate nutritional repletion. Which of the following statements is true regarding postoperative nutrition?

a. Enteral nutrition has no advantages over parenteral nutrition in postoperative patients.
b. Institution of enteral feeding within 24 hours postoperatively is safe.
c. Institution of enteral feeding should be delayed until bowel function returns as evidenced by passage of flatus or a bowel movement.
d. Parenteral nutrition should be instituted immediately postoperatively and continued until enteral feeds have been initiated.
e. Return of gastric motility postoperatively occurs before return of small-bowel motility.

6-33. A 60-year-old man with known hepatitis C and a previous liver biopsy showing cirrhosis requests evaluation for possible liver transplantation. He has never received treatment for hepatitis C. Though previously a heavy user of alcohol, he has been abstinent for over 2 years. He has had 2 episodes of bleeding esophageal varices. He was hospitalized 6 months ago with acute hepatic encephalopathy. He has a 1 year history of ascites that has required repeated paracentesis despite treatment with diuretics.

Medications are aldactone 100 mg daily and lactulose 30 cc 3 times daily.

On examination he appears thin, with obvious scleral icterus, spider angiomas, palmar erythema, gynecomastia, a large amount ascites, and small testicles. There is no asterixis.

Recent laboratory testing revealed the following: hemoglobin = 12.0 mg/dL (normal 13.5-15.0), MCV = 103 fL (normal 80-100), creatinine = 2.0 mg/dL (normal 0.7-1.2), bilirubin = 6.5 mg/dL (normal 0.1-1.2), AST = 25 U/L (normal< 40), ALT = 45 U/L (normal < 40), INR = 3.0 (normal 0.8-1.2).

What is the next best step?

a. Repeat liver biopsy.
b. Start treatment with interferon and ribavirin.
c. Refer the patient for hospice care.
d. Continue to optimize medical treatment for his ascites and hepatic encephalopathy and tell the patient he is not eligible for liver transplantation because of his previous history of alcohol abuse.
e. Refer the patient to a liver transplantation center.

6-34. A 26-year-old woman with panic disorder notes that during the middle of one of her attacks she feels as if she is disconnected from the world, as though it were unreal or distant. Which of the following terms best describes this symptom?

a. Mental status change
b. Illusion
c. Retardation of thought
d. Depersonalization
e. Derealization

6-35. A 51-year-old woman presents to the ED after 5 consecutive days of crushing substernal chest pressure that woke her up from sleep in the morning. The pain resolves spontaneously after 20 to 30 minutes. She is an avid rock climber and jogs 5 miles daily. She has never smoked cigarettes and has no family history of coronary disease. In the ED, she experiences another episode of chest pain. An ECG reveals ST-segment elevations and cardiac biomarkers are negative. The pain is relieved with sublingual nitroglycerin. She is admitted to the hospital and diagnostic testing reveals minimal coronary atherosclerotic disease. Which of the following is the most appropriate medication to treat this patient's condition?

a. Aspirin
b. Calcium channel blocker (CCB)
c. β-Blocker
d. H$_2$-Blocker
e. Antidepressant

6-36. A 38-year-old man comes to the office to discuss his headache symptoms. He describes the headaches as severe and intense, "like an ice pick in my eye!" The headaches begin suddenly, are unilateral, last up to 2 hours, and are associated with a runny nose and watery eye on the affected side. He gets several attacks over a couple of months, but is symptom-free for months in-between flare ups. Which of the following is the best approach for prophylactic management of the attacks?

a. SSRIs
b. Triptans
c. NSAIDs
d. Calcium channel blockers
e. Ergotamine

6-37. A 76-year-old woman presents with acute onset of persistent back pain and hypotension. A CT scan is obtained (shown below), and the patient is taken emergently to the operating room. Three days after surgery she complains of abdominal pain and bloody mucus per rectum. Which of the following is the most likely diagnosis?

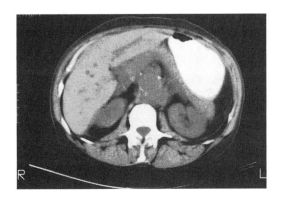

a. Staphylococcal enterocolitis
b. Diverticulitis
c. Bleeding arteriovenous (AV) malformation
d. Ischemia of the left colon
e. Bleeding colonic carcinoma

6-38. A 17-year-old boy is brought to the emergency department by his parents with the complaint of coughing up blood. He is stabilized, and his hemoglobin and hematocrit levels are 11 mg/dL and 33%, respectively. During his hospitalization, he is noted to have systolic blood pressure persistently greater than 130 mm Hg and diastolic blood pressure greater than 90 mm Hg. His urinalysis is remarkable for hematuria and proteinuria. You are suspicious the patient has which of the following?

a. Hemolytic-uremic syndrome
b. Goodpasture syndrome
c. Nephrotic syndrome
d. Poststreptococcal glomerulonephritis
e. Renal vein thrombosis

Questions 39 to 43

Match each description with the correct type of abortion. Each lettered option may be used once, more than once, or not at all.

a. Complete abortion
b. Incomplete abortion
c. Threatened abortion
d. Missed abortion
e. Inevitable abortion

6-39. Uterine bleeding at 12 weeks gestation accompanied by cervical dilation without passage of tissue.

6-40. Passage of some but not all placental tissue through the cervix at 9 weeks gestation.

6-41. Fetal death at 15 weeks gestation without expulsion of any fetal or maternal tissue for at least 8 weeks.

6-42. Uterine bleeding at 7 weeks gestation without any cervical dilation.

6-43. Expulsion of all fetal and placental tissue from the uterine cavity at 10 weeks gestation.

6-44. A 19-year-old male college student returns from spring break in Fort Lauderdale, Florida, with complaints of acute pain and swelling of the scrotum. Physical examination reveals an exquisitely tender, swollen right testis that is rather hard to examine. The cremasteric reflex is absent, but there is no swelling in the inguinal area. The rest of his genitourinary examination appears to be normal. A urine dip is negative for red and white blood cells. Which of the following is the appropriate next step in management?

a. Administration of antibiotics after culture of urethra for *Chlamydia* and gonorrhea
b. Reassurance
c. Intravenous fluid administration, pain medications, and straining of all voids
d. Ultrasound of the scrotum
e. Laparoscopic exploration of both inguinal regions

6-45. A 72-year-old male with a history of poorly controlled hypertension develops a viral upper respiratory infection. On his second day of symptoms he experiences palpitations and presents to the emergency room. His blood pressure is 118/78. The following rhythm strip is obtained. What is the best next step in the management of this patient?

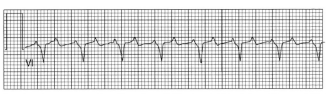

(Reproduced, with permission, from Fauci A et al. Harrison's Principles of Internal Medicine, 17th ed. New York, NY: McGraw-Hill, 2008.)

a. Administration of intravenous metoprolol
b. Administration of intravenous adenosine
c. Administration of intravenous amiodarone
d. Emergent electrical cardioversion
e. Initiation of chest compressions and preparation for semielective intubation

6-46. A 78-year-old man complains of increasing fatigue and bone pain, especially around the knees and ankles. He has been anemic for several years, with hemoglobin of 9 to 10 g/dL and MCV of 102. His leukocyte and platelet count have been normal; he has not had lymphadenopathy or splenomegaly. He had not responded to therapeutic trials of iron and vitamin B_{12}, but has been symptomatically stable until the past month. Examination reveals pallor and spleen tip at the left costal margin. CBC reveals hemoglobin of 8.2 g/dL, but for the first time his platelet count is low (15,000); the white blood cell count is 14,000. What is the likely cause of his worsening anemia?

a. Folic acid deficiency
b. Acute myeloid leukemia
c. Myelofibrosis
d. Tuberculosis
e. Viral infection

Block 7

Questions

7-1. A 5-year-old boy shows no interest in other children and ignores adults other than his parents. He spends hours lining up his toy cars or spinning their wheels but does not use them for "make-believe" play. He rarely uses speech to communicate, and his parents state that he has never done so. Physical examination indicates that his head is of normal circumference and his gait is normal. Which of the following is the most likely diagnosis for this boy?

a. Obsessive-compulsive disorder
b. Asperger syndrome
c. Childhood disintegrative disorder
d. Autism
e. Rett disorder

7-2. A 36-year-old woman comes to your office complaining of recurrent dysuria. This is her fourth episode in the past 10 months. Initially, her symptoms were "classic" for a UTI. She was treated without obtaining urine dipstick or microscopic evaluation. For the second episode, her urinalysis was positive for blood only. Her culture was negative, as was evaluation for nephrolithiasis. The third episode was similar, also with a negative culture. All episodes have resolved with a standard course of antibiotic therapy. Which of the following is the most appropriate next step?

a. Evaluate for somatization disorder
b. Order cystoscopy
c. Treat for chronic vaginitis
d. Use a 14-day regimen of antibiotics
e. Use daily single-dose antibiotic therapy for prophylaxis

7-3. A 78-year-old woman is referred to a neurologist for evaluation of a tremor. She says that it is not very bothersome to her, but others have noticed it. It primarily involves the right hand and apparently has been slowly worsening over the past 12 to 18 months. Examination reveals a resting tremor of the right upper extremity, accompanied by mild rigidity and slowness of rapid alternating movements. Which of the following medications is the best choice to treat the symptoms of this disease?

a. Alteplase
b. Carbidopa-levodopa
c. Glatiramer
d. Interferon β-1A
e. Sertraline

7-4. A 53-year-old woman presents with increasing weakness, most noticeable in the legs. She has noticed some cramping and weakness in the upper extremities as well. She has more difficulty removing the lids from jars than before. She has noticed some stiffness in the neck but denies back pain or injury. There is no bowel or bladder incontinence. She takes naproxen for osteoarthritis and is on alendronate for osteoporosis. She smokes one pack of cigarettes daily. The general physical examination reveals decreased range of motion in the cervical spine. On neurological examination, the patient has 4/5 strength in the hands with mild atrophy of the interosseous muscles. She also has 4/5 strength in the feet; the weakness is more prominent in the distal musculature. She has difficulty with both heel walking and toe walking. Reflexes are hyperactive in the lower extremities. Sustained clonus is demonstrated at the ankles. What is the best next step in her management?

a. Obtain MRI scan of the head
b. Begin riluzole
c. Obtain MRI scan of the cervical spine
d. Check muscle enzymes including creatine kinase and aldolase
e. Refer for physical therapy and gait training exercises

7-5. A 64-year-old woman presents with diffuse hair loss. She says that her hair is "coming out by the handfuls" after shampooing. She was treated for severe community-acquired pneumonia 2 months ago but has regained her strength and is exercising regularly. She is taking no medications. Examination reveals diffuse hair loss. Several hairs can be removed by gentle tugging. The scalp is normal without scale or erythema. Her general examination is unremarkable; in particular, her vital signs are normal, she has no pallor or inflammatory synovitis, and her reflexes are normal with a normal relaxation phase. What is the best next step in her management?

a. Reassurance
b. Measurement of serum testosterone and DHEA-S levels
c. Topical minoxidil
d. Topical corticosteroids
e. CBC and antinuclear antibodies

7-6. A 23-year-old woman comes to the physician with the chief complaint of a depressed mood for 6 months. She states that she has felt lethargic, does not sleep well, and has decreased energy and difficulty concentrating. She notes that she has gained over 15 lb without attempting to do so, and seems to bruise much more easily than previously. On physical examination, she is noted to have numerous purple striae on her abdomen, proximal muscle weakness, and a loss of peripheral vision. A brain tumor is found on MRI. In which of the following areas of the brain was this tumor most likely found?

a. Frontal lobe
b. Cerebellum
c. Thalamus
d. Pituitary
e. Brainstem

7-7. A 24-year-old woman presents with lethargy, anorexia, tachypnea, and weakness. Laboratory studies reveal a BUN of 150 mg/dL, serum creatinine of 16 mg/dL, and potassium of 6.2 mEq/L. Chest x-ray shows increased pulmonary vascularity and a dilated heart. Which of the following is the most appropriate management of this patient?

a.   Emergency kidney transplantation
b.   Creation and immediate use of a forearm arteriovenous fistula
c.   Placement of a catheter in the internal jugular vein and initiation of hemodialysis
d.   A 100-g protein diet
e.   Renal biopsy

7-8. A 57-year-old man has been having nightly, unilateral, throbbing headaches. They have been occurring daily for the past week. The patient recalls having had a similar headache 5 years ago that lasted for several weeks. The patient has noticed that the headache is associated with lacrimation and a "stuffy nose." Ergotamine prophylaxis has been partially successful. Which of the following is the most effective means of aborting this type of headache?

a.   Inhaled 100% oxygen
b.   Sublingual nitroglycerin
c.   Oral methysergide
d.   Oral propranolol
e.   Dihydroergotamine suppository

Questions 9 to 10

7-9. A 40-year-old woman is brought to the ED by the paramedics complaining of bilateral foot weakness and numbness that started a few hours ago and is progressively worsening. She denies similar episodes in the past. On the review of systems, she describes having abdominal cramps with nausea, vomiting, and diarrhea 2 weeks ago that resolved after 2 to 3 days. Her BP is 124/67 mm Hg, HR is 68 beats per minute, temperature is 98.8°F, and RR is 12 breaths per minute. On examination, you elicit 2/5 strength, decreased sensation, and loss of deep tendon reflexes in the lower extremities below the hips. Which of the following is the most likely diagnosis?

a.   Hypokalemic periodic paralysis
b.   Guillain-Barré syndrome
c.   Peripheral vascular disease
d.   Tetanus
e.   Brain abscess

7-10. What life-threatening complication is associated with this disease process described in the previous question?

a. Permanent paralysis
b. Thrombocytopenia
c. Respiratory failure
d. Need for surgery
e. Kidney failure

7-11. A 16-year-old girl presents with lower abdominal pain and fever. On physical examination, a tender adnexal mass is felt. Further questioning in private reveals the following: she has a new sexual partner; her periods are irregular; she has a vaginal discharge. Which of the following is the most likely diagnosis?

a. Appendiceal abscess
b. Tubo-ovarian abscess
c. Ovarian cyst
d. Renal cyst
e. Ectopic pregnancy

7-12. A 57-year-old man is seeing a psychiatrist for the treatment of his major depression. During the course of his treatment, the man describes in great detail the fact that he has molested several children. Some of these molestations occurred decades previously, but one, according to the patient, is ongoing, involving a 10-year-old boy who lives in an apartment next door to the patient. Which of the following actions should the psychiatrist take next?

a. The psychiatrist should take no action outside the therapeutic setting but, rather, try to explore the unconscious determinants of this patient's behavior.
b. The psychiatrist should take no action outside the therapeutic setting because the patient is protected by confidentiality laws.
c. The psychiatrist should admit the patient to a psychiatric hospital and call the boy's parents to alert them to the danger.
d. The psychiatrist should call the police and have them apprehend the patient at the next treatment session.
e. The psychiatrist should immediately report the patient's behavior to the appropriate state agency.

7-13. A 75-year-old woman is accompanied by her daughter to your clinic. The daughter reports that her mother fell in her yard last week while watering flowers. Her mother suffered scratches and bruises but no serious injury. The daughter is concerned that her mother might fall again with serious injury. The patient has hypertension and osteoarthritis of the knees. She takes HCTZ, lisinopril, naproxen, and occasional diphenhydramine for sleep. The daughter reports some mild forgetfulness over the past 2 years. The patient gets up frequently at night to urinate.

Blood pressure is 142/78 lying and 136/74 standing. Pulse is 64 lying and standing. Except for some patellofemoral crepitance of the knees, her physical examination is normal. A Folstein mini-mental status testing is normal except that she only remembers two of three objects after 3 minutes (29/30). She takes 14 seconds to rise from sitting in a hard backed chair, walk 10 ft, turn, return to the chair, and sit down (timed up-and-go test, normal less than 10 seconds). A CBC, chemistry profile, and thyroid tests are normal.

What is the next best step?

a. CT scan of the brain
b. Holter monitor
c. Discontinue hydrochlorothiazide and prescribe donepezil
d. Discontinue diphenhydramine, assess her home for fall risks, and prescribe physical therapy
e. EEG

7-14. A 60-year-old otherwise healthy woman presents to her physician with a 3-week history of severe headaches. A contrast CT scan reveals a small, circular, hypodense lesion with ringlike contrast enhancement. Which of the following is the most likely diagnosis?

a. Brain abscess
b. High-grade astrocytoma
c. Parenchymal hemorrhage
d. Metastatic lesion
e. Toxoplasmosis

7-15. You are caring for a 45-year-old man with fatigue. Workup revealed hereditary hemochromatosis, an autosomal recessive disorder. Neither of his parents ever showed signs of the disease, though they were never tested while alive. Your patient has one sister. What is the chance that his sister is affected?

a. No chance
b. 10% chance
c. 25% chance
d. 50% chance
e. 100% chance

7-16. A 4-year-old boy presents with a history of constipation since the age of 6 months. His stools, produced every 3 to 4 days, are described as large and hard. Physical examination is normal; rectal examination reveals a large ampulla, poor sphincter tone but present anal wink, and stool in the rectal vault. The plain film of his abdomen is shown. Which of the following is the most appropriate next step in the management of this child?

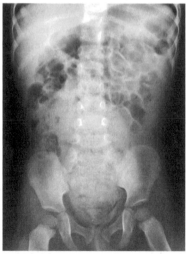

(Used with permission from Susan John, MD.)

a. Lower gastrointestinal (GI) barium study
b. Parental reassurance and dietary counseling
c. Serum electrolyte measurement
d. Upper GI barium study
e. Initiation of thyroid-replacement hormone

7-17. A 45-year-old right-handed man who has been HIV positive for the past 3 years has noticed some sort of visual change over the past 1 to 2 months. It is difficult for him to describe, but it is some sort of distortion of part of his right visual field. There is a 4-cm rim-enhancing lesion in the left occipital lobe that is revealed by MRI. Which of the following tumor types is common in the brain of patients with AIDS, but otherwise extremely rare?

a. Lymphocytic leukemia
b. Metastatic lymphoma
c. Primary lymphoma
d. Kaposi sarcoma
e. Lymphosarcoma

7-18. A 42-year-old man sees you because of obesity. He played football in high school and at age 18 weighed 250 pounds. He has gradually gained weight since. Many previous attempts at dieting have resulted in transient weight loss of 10 to 15 pounds, which he then rapidly regains. He has been attending Weight Watchers for the last 3 months and has successfully lost 4 pounds. Recent attempts at exercise have been limited because of bilateral knee pain and swelling. On examination height is 6 ft 0 in, weight 340 pounds, BMI 46. Blood pressure with a large cuff is 150/95. Baseline laboratory studies including CBC, biochemical profile, thyroid stimulating hormone and lipids are normal with the exception of fasting serum glucose which is 145 mg/dL. What is the next best step?

a. Discuss bariatric surgery with the patient.
b. Refer to a commercial weight-loss program.
c. Recommend a 1000 calorie per day diet.
d. Prescribe sibutramine.
e. Recommend a low-fat diet.

7-19. A patient is noted incidentally on an ultrasound to have a right renal mass. Which of the following statements is true regarding further workup and treatment of a renal mass?

a. Presence of a simple cyst requires follow-up imaging in a year.
b. Diagnosis of an angiomyolipoma of the kidney requires surgical resection.
c. Presence of a 3-cm lesion suspicious for renal cell carcinoma can be treated with a partial nephrectomy.
d. Computed tomographic (CT) scanning is diagnostic for oncocytomas.
e. Presence of a solid, enhancing lesion in the right kidney should always be biopsied percutaneously.

7-20. A 28-year-old woman is seen for postpartum blues by the psychiatrist. She states she is depressed because she "did this to her child." The infant has growth retardation, microphthalmia, short palpebral fissures, midface hypoplasia, a short philtrum, a thin upper lip, and microcephaly. Which is the most likely diagnosis of the mother (besides the postpartum blues)?

a. Bipolar disorder
b. Major depression
c. Hypochondriasis
d. Alcohol dependence
e. Cocaine dependence

7-21. A 56-year-old woman with a history of ovarian cancer presents to the ED with acute onset of right-sided chest pain, shortness of breath, and dyspnea. Her BP is 131/75 mm Hg, HR is 101 beats per minute, respirations are 18 breaths per minute, and oxygen saturation is 97% on room air. You suspect this patient has a pulmonary embolism (PE). Which of the following tests is most likely to be abnormal?

a. Arterial blood gas
b. Oxygen saturation
c. ECG
d. Chest radiograph
e. D-dimer

7-22. A 69-year-old man with mild hypertension and chronic obstructive pulmonary disease (COPD) presents with transient ischemic attacks and the angiogram shown here. Which of the following is the most appropriate treatment recommendation?

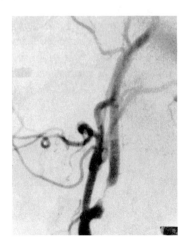

a. Medical therapy with aspirin 325 mg/day and medical risk factor management
b. Medical therapy with warfarin
c. Angioplasty of the carotid lesion followed by carotid endarterectomy if the angioplasty is unsuccessful
d. Carotid endarterectomy
e. Medical risk factor management and carotid endarterectomy if neurologic symptoms develop

7-23. You are caring for a 42-year-old woman who was diagnosed with rheumatoid arthritis (RA) 8 years ago. You are concerned about potential extra-articular manifestations of her disease. Which of the following signs or symptoms, if present, would signal extra-articular manifestations RA?

a. Cough
b. Congestive heart failure (CHF)
c. Gastrointestinal (GI) distress
d. Peripheral neuropathy
e. Renal failure

7-24. A 28-year-old nonsmoking woman presents to discuss birth control methods. She requests a contraceptive option that is not associated with weight gain. She and her husband agree that they desire no children for the next few years. Her periods are regular, but heavy and painful. She frequently stays home from work on the first day due to severe lower abdominal cramping and back pain. She changes her pad every 4 hours. This pattern of bleeding has been present since she was 15 years old. For a week before her period begins, she is uncharacteristically tearful, irritable, and depressed. Her behavior change before her period is beginning to affect her work relationships. Her physical examination reveals blood pressure 110/75, BMI 22, and moderate acne on her face and neck. What recommendation will best address her mood, skin, and contraceptive needs?

a. Tubal ligation
b. Drosperinone and estrogen combination pill
c. Progesterone-infused intrauterine device
d. Progesterone shots every 3 months
e. Condoms

7-25. A father brings his 3-year-old daughter to the emergency center after noting her to be pale and tired and with a subjective fever for several days. Her past history is significant for an upper respiratory infection 4 weeks prior, but she had been otherwise healthy. The father denies emesis or diarrhea, but does report his daughter has had leg pain over the previous week, waking her from sleep. He also reports that she has been bleeding from her gums after brushing her teeth. Examination reveals a listless pale child. She has diffuse lymphadenopathy with splenomegaly but no hepatomegaly. She has a few petechiae scattered across her face and abdomen and is mildly tender over her shins, but does not have associated erythema or joint swelling. A CBC reveals a leukocyte count of 8,000/μL with a hemoglobin of 4 g/dL and a platelet count of 7,000/μL. The automated differential reports an elevated number of atypical lymphocytes. Which of the following diagnostic studies is the most appropriate next step in the management of this child?

a. Epstein-Barr virus titers
b. Serum haptoglobin
c. Antiplatelet antibody assay
d. Reticulocyte count
e. Bone marrow biopsy

7-26. A 32-year-old woman reports that she sometimes "skips heartbeats." Her medical and social histories include moderate daily caffeine use, but are otherwise unremarkable. Her physical examination and 12-lead ECG are normal, as are her CBC, electrolytes, and TSH. Which of the following is the next appropriate step in her workup?

a. Reassure her and continue observation
b. Perform ambulatory ECG monitoring (a 24-Holter monitor, or a continuous loop event recorder)
c. Electrophysiology consultation
d. Stress testing
e. Echocardiography

7-27. A 20-month-old male infant is placed in an emergency department of children and family services shelter after his mother is hospitalized as the result of a car accident. Three days after the separation, the child spends almost every waking moment crying and calling and searching for his mother. The fourth day after the separation, when the mother of the child comes to the shelter to reclaim her child, he rejects her offers of affection, instead clinging to the nurse's aide who has been his caretaker. Which of the following terms most accurately describes this infant's reactions to a forced separation?

a. Protest
b. Despair
c. Detachment
d. Denial
e. Acting out

7-28. A 19-year-old man goes swimming in an inland pond in Puerto Rico. Within a few days, he notices itching of his skin over several surfaces of his body. He is unconcerned until several weeks later when he develops lancinating pains extending down his legs and all of his toes. Over the course of just a few days, he develops paraparesis and problems with bladder and bowel control. Within 1 week, he is unable to stand and has severe urinary retention. Which of the following is the most appropriate plan of action on an emergency basis?

a. Initiate anticoagulation
b. Perform sensory-evoked potential testing
c. Order an MRI scan
d. Place a cervical collar
e. Perform spinal angiography

7-29. A 43-year-old G2P2 comes to your office complaining of an intermittent right nipple discharge that is bloody. She reports that the discharge is spontaneous and not associated with any nipple pruritus, burning, or discomfort. On physical examination, you do not detect any dominant breast masses or adenopathy. There are no skin changes noted. Which of the following conditions is the most likely cause of this patient's problem?

a. Breast cancer
b. Duct ectasia
c. Intraductal papilloma
d. Fibrocystic breast disease
e. Pituitary adenoma

7-30. A 70-year-old man with diabetes and long-term osteoarthritis in his knees is presenting for follow-up. He reports that his pain has become much more severe, and says he is having difficulty with ambulation and is becoming fairly inactive. In the past, he tried ibuprofen and naproxen, but those offered limited improvement and he developed secondary ulcers. He says that taking acetaminophen is like "taking a sugar pill"—it offers no help. He had some relief from steroid injections 3 months ago, and again 1 month ago, but they were short-lived. A recent x-ray is shown below:

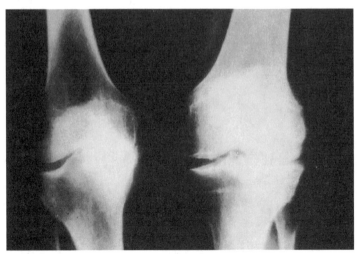

(Reproduced, with permission, from South-Paul J. Current Diagnosis and Treatment in Family Medicine, *1st ed. New York: McGraw-Hill, 2004:267.)*

Which of the following is the next most appropriate step in the treatment of his condition?

a. Use oral steroids
b. Try another steroid injection
c. Inject the knee joint with ketorolac (Toradol)
d. Inject hyaluronic acid into his knee joints
e. Refer for knee replacements

7-31. A 60-year-old asymptomatic man is found to have leukocytosis on a preoperative CBC. Physical examination shows the spleen tip to be palpable 2 cm below the left costal margin. Rubbery, nontender lymph nodes up to 1.5 cm in size are present in the axillae and inguinal regions. Laboratory data include the following:

Hgb: 13.3 g/dL (normal 14 to 18)
Leukocytes: 40,000/μL (normal 4300 to 10,800)
Platelet count: 238,000 (normal 150,000 to 400,000)
His peripheral blood smear is shown in the accompanying photo.

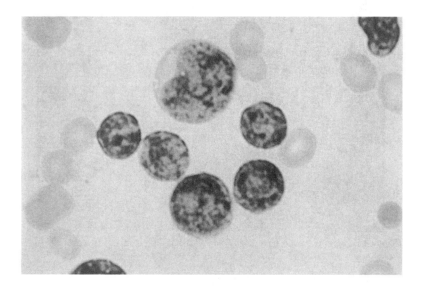

Which of the following is the most likely diagnosis?
a. Acute monocytic leukemia
b. Chronic myelogenous leukemia
c. Chronic lymphocytic leukemia
d. Tuberculosis
e. Infectious mononucleosis

7-32. A 52-year-old woman presented to the emergency room with a new-onset aphasia. A hemorrhagic left frontal mass is apparent on head CT. The neurosurgical consultant decides to explore the site of the hemorrhage and evacuate the mass that has collected there. He sends tissue from the margin of the blood clot for a frozen section analysis by the pathologist. The tissue is felt to be Kernohan grade IV astrocytoma. Which of the following post-operative therapies is most reasonable?

a. Cranial radiotherapy
b. Intravenous methotrexate
c. Intravenous fludarabine
d. Intravenous cyclophosphamide
e. Intravenous daunorubicin

Questions 33 to 36

Match the correct substance with the questions below. Each lettered option may be used once, more than once, or not at all.

a. Neuropeptide Y
b. GABA
c. Norepinephrine
d. Somatostatin
e. Substance P
f. Glutamate
g. Acetylcholine
h. Serotonin

7-33. Which of these substances is primarily affected by fluoxetine?

7-34. Which of these substances is most associated with the classic anti-depressant drugs, as well as venlafaxine, mirtazapine, and bupropion?

7-35. Which of these substances is most prominently associated with the mediation of the perception of pain?

7-36. Which of these substances has been shown to stimulate the appetite?

7-37. The developmentally delayed 6-month-old child in the picture below had intrauterine growth retardation (including microcephaly), hepatospleno-megaly, prolonged neonatal jaundice, and purpura at birth. The calcific densities in the skull x-ray shown are likely the result of which of the following?

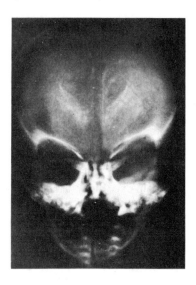

a. Congenital cytomegalovirus (CMV) infection
b. Congenital toxoplasmosis infection
c. Congenital syphilis infection
d. Tuberculous meningitis
e. Craniopharyngioma

7-38. A 58-year-old man presents to the ED with progressive dyspnea over the course of 1 week. Upon arrival, he is able to speak in full sentences and states that he stopped taking all of his medications recently. Initial vitals include a HR of 92 beats per minute, a BP of 180/100 mm Hg, and an RR of 16 breaths per minute with an oxygen saturation of 94% on room air. Upon physical examination, the patient has bibasilar crackles, jugular venous distention, and pedal edema. Which of the following medication regimens was the patient most likely on?

a. Loop diuretic only
b. Aspirin only
c. Loop diuretic and β-blocker
d. Calcium channel blocker
e. Loop diuretic, β-blocker, and angiotensin-converting enzyme (ACE) inhibitor

7-39. A 32-year-old woman presents to the ED with a 1-month history of general malaise, mild cough, and subjective fevers. She states that she is human immunodeficiency virus (HIV) positive and her last CD4 count, 6 months ago, was 220. She is not on antiretroviral therapy or any other medications. Initial vitals include a HR of 88 beats per minute, a BP of 130/60 mm Hg, and an RR of 12 breaths per minute with an oxygen saturation of 91% on room air. Her chest radiograph shows bilateral diffuse interstitial infiltrates. Subsequent laboratory tests are unremarkable except for an elevated lactate dehydrogenase level. Given this patient's history and physical examination, which of the following is the most likely organism responsible for her clinical presentation?

a. *Coccidioides immitis*
b. *Mycobacterium tuberculosis*
c. *Pneumocystis jiroveci*
d. *Mycoplasma pneumoniae*
e. *Haemophilus influenzae*

7-40. A 2-year-old boy is brought into the emergency room with a complaint of fever for 6 days and the development of a limp. On examination, he is found to have an erythematous macular exanthem over his body as shown in image A, ocular conjunctivitis, dry and cracked lips, a red throat, and cervical lymphadenopathy. There is a grade 2/6 vibratory systolic ejection murmur at the lower left sternal border. A white blood cell (WBC) count and differential show predominant neutrophils with increased platelets on smear. Later, he develops the findings as seen in image B. Which of the following is the most likely diagnosis?

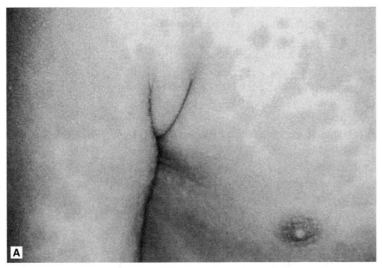

(Reproduced with permission from Wolff K, Johnson RA, Suurmond D. Fitzpatick's Color Atlas & Synopsis of Clinical Dermatology. 5th ed. New York, NY: McGraw-Hill; 2005.)

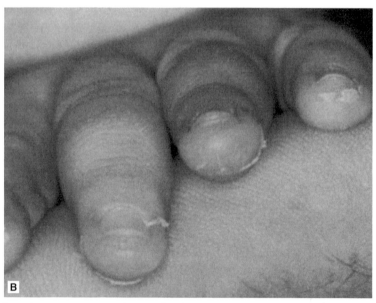

a. Scarlet fever
b. Rheumatic fever
c. Kawasaki disease
d. Juvenile rheumatoid arthritis
e. Infectious mononucleosis

7-41. A 65-year-old man develops a severe headache and right-sided weakness. He has a history of osteoarthritis, gout, and hypertension. He regularly keeps his follow-up visits and is compliant with his medications, which include lisinopril 10 mg po q AM for hypertension, allopurinol 300 mg po q AM to prevent gout, and acetaminophen for his joint pains. Review of his recent office record shows that his mean blood pressure has been 124/78. On physical examination the patient is drowsy but arousable. His blood pressure is 164/90 and his pulse rate is 56. He has a right homonymous hemianopsia and a mild right hemiparesis. Sensory examination is difficult due to poor cooperation. Cardiac examination shows no S_3 or S_4 gallop and a regular rhythm. He has no ecchymoses or evidence of abnormal bruising. His ECG is normal without left ventricular hypertrophy. CT of the head without IV contrast shows an acute hemorrhage in the left parietal lobe; the basal ganglia and thalamus are uninvolved. What is the likely pathogenesis of the neurological problem?

a. Small vessel vasculitis
b. Intimal damage to penetrating cerebral vessels
c. Trauma from domestic abuse
d. Coagulopathy
e. Amyloid deposition in the cerebral vasculature

Questions 42 to 46

Match each description with the appropriate fetal heart rate tracing. If none of the tracings apply, answer e (none). Each lettered option may be used once, more than once, or not at all.

a.

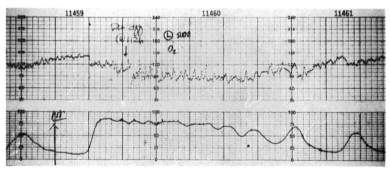

b.

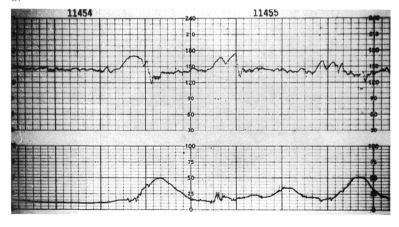

c.

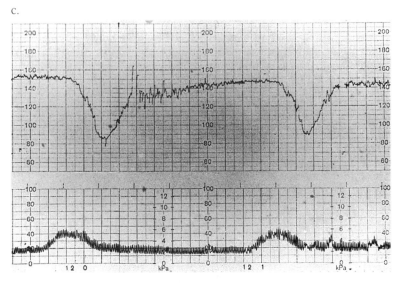

d.

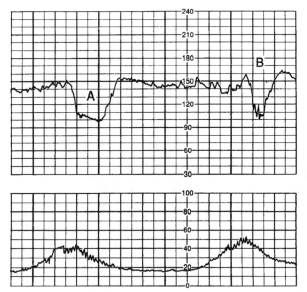

(Reproduced, with permission from: Cunningham FG, Leveno KL, Bloom SL, et al. Williams Obstetrics, 22nd ed., New York, McGraw-Hill, 2005, p. 455.)

e. None

7-42. A 23-year-old G1P0 at 42 weeks is undergoing induction of labor. She is receiving intravenous oxytocin. She complains that her contractions are very painful and seem to be continuous.

7-43. A laboring patient has an internal fetal scalp electrode in place. Pelvic examination shows the patient to be 7 cm dilated with the fetal vertex at +1 station. The fetal heart rate tracing is consistent with fetal head compression.

7-44. A patient at 41 weeks is undergoing NST. Her NST is reactive and reassuring.

7-45. A laboring patient at 40 weeks gestation presents with spontaneous rupture of membranes. Bedside ultrasonography shows no measurable pockets of amniotic fluid. With each contraction, the fetal heart rate tracing shows evidence of umbilical cord compression.

7-46. A preeclamptic patient at 33 weeks gestation with IUGR is undergoing induction of labor. The fetal heart rate tracing shows evidence of uteroplacental insufficiency and is nonreassuring.

Block 8

Questions

8-1. An 88-year-old resident of a local nursing home is transferred to your facility with shortness of breath. She has been coughing for the past 2 to 3 days. The patient has a history of mild dementia, but has had no witnessed episodes of coughing or choking when eating. Vital signs include a heart rate of 103/minute, respiratory rate of 22/minute, blood pressure 158/68 mm Hg, temperature of 37.9°C (100.2°F) with a weight of 52 kg. Upon examination, she is pleasant but disoriented. Chest auscultation reveals crackles in the left lower lung field. WBC count is 11,000, BUN is 32, and creatinine is 1.3. Chest radiograph shows an infiltrate in the left lower lobe, and induced sputum sample has been sent for Gram stain and culture. What is the best initial course of therapy for this patient?

a. Begin a third-generation cephalosporin and macrolide and admit her to the hospital.
b. Begin a renal-dosed third-generation cephalosporin and macrolide and admit her to the hospital.
c. Begin a respiratory fluoroquinolone and discharge her to the nursing home for follow-up.
d. Begin an antipseudomonal carbapenem, antipseudomonal respiratory fluoroquinolone, and glycopeptide and admit her to the hospital.
e. Begin a renal-dosed antipseudomonal carbapenem, antipseudomonal respiratory fluoroquinolone, and glycopeptide and admit her to the hospital.

8-2. A patient reports horizontal double vision. When a red glass is placed over her right eye and she is asked to look at a flashlight off to her left, she reports seeing a white light and a red light. The red light appears to her to be more to the left than the white light. Her right pupil is more dilated than her left pupil and responds less briskly to a bright light directed at it than does the left pupil. The injury likely to be responsible for all of these observations is one involving which of the following nerves?

a. The second cranial nerve
b. The third cranial nerve
c. The fourth cranial nerve
d. The sixth cranial nerve
e. None of the above

8-3. A 30-year-old woman presents to the psychiatrist with a 2 month history of difficulty in concentrating, irritability, and depression. She has never had these symptoms before. Three months prior to her visit to the psychiatrist, the patient noted that she had experienced a short-lived flu-like illness with a rash on her calf, but has noted no other symptoms since then until the mood symptoms began. Her physical examination was within normal limits. Which of the following is the most likely diagnosis?

a. Neurosyphilis
b. Chronic meningitis
c. Lyme disease
d. Creutzfeldt-Jakob disease
e. Prion disease

8-4. A 60-year-old, right-handed man presents with visual loss. About 2 weeks before, he began to notice difficulty seeing the television. Within 1 week, he noticed that the inferior field of vision in the right eye was much worse than the top of his vision. Within a few more days, he noticed the bottom of the vision in his left eye worsen as well. This has been painless. He has otherwise felt well, without headaches or cognitive changes. An ophthalmologist saw bilateral papillitis with white exudates of the nasal part of the discs. There is no history of alcohol use, and the patient has stopped smoking since his heart transplant. On examination, he appears well. Blood pressure is 160/80 mm Hg; pulse is 100 beats per minute and regular. There are no carotid bruits. Pupils are equal and reactive. Visual acuity is 20/400 OU, with central-inferior scotomas (left larger than right). Neurologic examination is otherwise normal. An MRI scan with and without gadolinium contrast agent, including orbital cuts, is negative, as is CSF examination. This patient's history, examination, and laboratory findings are now most consistent with which of the following diagnoses?

a. Cyclosporine toxicity
b. Occipital lobe lymphoma
c. Tobacco-alcohol amblyopia
d. Ischemic optic neuropathies
e. Retinal detachment

8-5. An 18-year-old woman is brought to the ED by her mother. The patient is diaphoretic and vomiting. Her mom states that she thinks her daughter tried to commit suicide. The patient admits to ingesting a few handfuls of extra-strength Tylenol approximately 3 hours ago. Her temperature is 99.1°F, BP is 105/70 mm Hg, HR is 92 beats per minute, RR is 17 breaths per minute, and oxygen saturation is 99% on room air. On examination, her head and neck are unremarkable. Cardiovascular and pulmonary examinations are within normal limits. She is mildly tender in her right upper quadrant but there is no rebound or guarding. Bowel sounds are normoactive. She is alert and oriented and has no focal deficits on neurologic examination. You administer 50 g of activated charcoal. At this point, she appears well and has no complaints. Her 4-hour serum acetaminophen (APAP) concentration returns at 350 μg/mL. You plot the level on the nomogram seen below. Which of the following is the most appropriate next step in management?

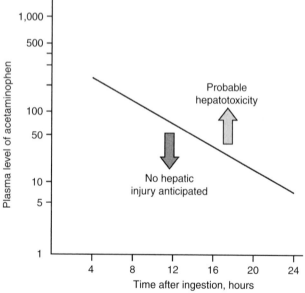

(Reproduced, with permission, from Brunton LL et al. Goodman and Gilman's The Pharmacological Basis Therapeutics. New York, NY: McGraw-Hill, 2006: 694.)

a. Discharge home with instructions to return if symptoms return
b. Observe for 6 hours and if the patient still has no complaints discharge her home
c. Admit to the hospital for serial abdominal examinations
d. Admit to the psychiatry unit and keep on suicide watch while performing serial abdominal examinations
e. Begin NAC and admit to the hospital

8-6. A 46-year-old woman presents to the ED with her husband complaining of flu-like symptoms, headache, vomiting, and dyspnea. She states that she never had similar symptoms in the past and that her husband is getting sick with similar symptoms as well but refuses to see a doctor. She reports feeling well yesterday and even helped her husband set up a home generator in their garage. Her BP is 142/85 mm Hg, HR is 97 beats per minute, temperature is 100.6°F, and RR is 20 breaths per minute. On examination the patient is slow to respond to questions. Which of the following is the most appropriate diagnostic test?

a. Send blood to check the white blood cell (WBC) count.
b. Order a head CT scan.
c. Send blood to check the carboxyhemoglobin level.
d. Perform an LP.
e. No testing is necessary at this point.

8-7. The left ureter is partially transected (50% of circumference) during the course of a difficult operation on an unstable, critically ill patient. Which of the following would be the most appropriate management of this injury given the patient's unstable condition?

a. Placement of an external stent through the proximal ureteral stump with delayed reconstruction
b. Ipsilateral nephrectomy
c. Placement of a catheter from the distal ureter through an abdominal wall stab wound
d. Placement of a closed suction drain adjacent to the injury
e. Bringing the proximal ureter up to the skin as a ureterostomy

8-8. A mother brings her daughter in to see you for consultation. The daughter is 17 years old and has not started her period. She is 4 ft 10 in tall. She has no breast budding. On pelvic examination, she has no pubic hair. By digital examination, the patient has a cervix and uterus. The ovaries are not palpable. As part of the workup, serum FSH and LH levels are drawn and both are high. Which of the following is the most likely reason for delayed puberty and sexual infantilism in this patient?

a. Adrenogenital syndrome (testicular feminization)
b. McCune-Albright syndrome
c. Kallmann syndrome
d. Gonadal dysgenesis
e. Müllerian agenesis

8-9. A 65-year-old woman lives alone in a dilapidated house, although her family members have tried in vain to move her to a better dwelling. She wears odd and out-of-fashion clothes and rummages in the garbage cans of her neighbors to look for redeemable cans and bottles. She is very suspicious of her neighbors. She was convinced that her neighbors were plotting against her life for a brief time after she was mugged and thrown onto the pavement by a teenager, but now thinks that this is not the case. She believes in the "power of crystals to protect me" and has them strewn haphazardly throughout her house. Which of the following is the most likely diagnosis?

a. Autism
b. Schizophrenia, paranoid type
c. Schizotypal personality disorder
d. Avoidant personality disorder
e. Schizoid personality disorder

8-10. You are seeing a 34-year-old man with urinary symptoms. He reports frequency, urgency, and moderate back pain. He is febrile and acutely ill. He has no penile discharge. His urinalysis shows marked pyuria. He has never had an episode like this before, and has no known urinary tract abnormalities. Which of the following is the most likely diagnosis?

a. Gonococcal urethritis
b. Nongonococcal urethritis
c. Acute bacterial cystitis
d. Pyelonephritis
e. Acute prostatitis

8-11. A 32-year-old stockbroker sees you because she has felt anxious almost every day for the past 9 months. She feels "keyed up" at work. At times she has difficulty concentrating and has made several minor errors in clients' accounts. For the past year she has frequently had trouble falling asleep at night despite the fact that she always feels tired. She does not fall asleep during the day at inopportune times. She takes supplemental calcium but no other medications. She denies substance or alcohol abuse. Her vital signs and physical examination are normal. CBC and chemistry panel are normal. What is the most likely diagnosis?

a. Hyperthyroidism
b. Hyperparathyroidism
c. Generalized anxiety disorder
d. Obstructive sleep apnea
e. Frontal lobe dementia

8-12. A 4-week-old boy presents with a 10-day history of vomiting that has increased in frequency and forcefulness. The vomitus is not bile stained. The child feeds avidly and looks well, but he has been losing weight. An ultrasound of the abdomen is shown. Which of the following is the most likely diagnosis?

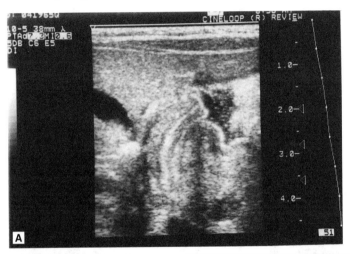

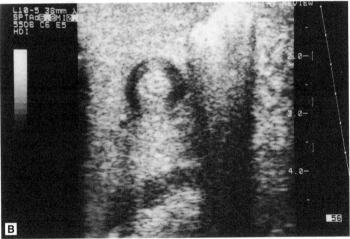

a. Surgical consultation for pyloromyotomy
b. Upper GI with small-bowel follow through
c. Intravenous (IV) fluids alone to maintain hydration
d. Air contrast enema
e. Computed tomography (CT) of the brain

8-13. A 37-year-old woman develops cholecystitis and requires cholecystectomy. Her family advises the physicians involved that she has a long history of alcoholism and benzodiazepine use, including diazepam (Valium), lorazepam (Ativan), and clonazepam (Klonopin). Approximately 7 days after the surgery, the patient becomes increasingly agitated, delusional, and suspicious. Routine investigations reveal no evidence of focal or systemic infection. Hepatic, renal, and hematologic parameters are largely normal. Within 24 hours of these cognitive and affective changes, the patient has a generalized tonic-clonic seizure. Magnetic resonance imaging (MRI) and computed tomography (CT) studies of the brain are normal, and her CSF is unremarkable. In consideration of the abuse history provided by the family, medication orders prior to the surgery should have included which of the following?

a. Haloperidol
b. Chlorpromazine
c. Trihexyphenidyl
d. Prochlorperazine
e. Thiamine

8-14. You are evaluating a 14-year-old girl with pelvic pain. She denies being sexually active and you do not suspect abuse. On pelvic examination, you confirm that she has never been sexually active, see no discharge and find no cervical motion tenderness, but feel an ovarian mass on the right side. Which of the following is the most appropriate next step in this situation?

a. Reassurance and use of NSAIDs for pain control
b. Reassurance and repeat pelvic examination in 6 to 8 weeks
c. Transvaginal pelvic ultrasound
d. CT scanning of the abdomen and pelvis
e. MRI evaluation of the pelvis

8-15. A 28-year-old man is brought to the ER for a severe head injury after a fall. He was intubated in the field for his decreased level of consciousness. He is tachycardic and hypotensive. On examination, he is noted to have an obvious skull fracture and his right pupil is dilated. Which of the following is the most appropriate method for initially reducing his intracranial pressure?

a. Elevation of the head of the bed
b. Saline-furosemide (Lasix) infusion
c. Mannitol infusion
d. Intravenous dexamethasone (Decadron)
e. Hyperventilation

8-16. An 82-year-old man presents to the ED feeling weak and dizzy. He has a past medical history of hypertension and diabetes and both are well controlled on hydrochlorothiazide, benazepril, atenolol, and metformin. On review of systems, he denies chest pain, gastrointestinal (GI) bleeding, and syncope, but states that he feels short of breath. His temperature is 98.6°F orally, BP is 86/60 mm Hg, HR is 44 beats per minute, RR is 18 breaths per minute, oxygen saturation is 98% on room air, and glucose is 116 mg/dL. He is immediately connected to the cardiac monitor. Which of the following choices best describes the ECG seen below?

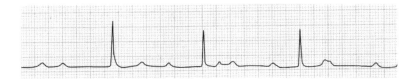

a. Normal sinus rhythm
b. First-degree AV block
c. Second-degree Mobitz I (Wenckebach) AV block
d. Second-degree Mobitz II AV block
e. Third-degree AV block

8-17. At the time of annual examination, a patient expresses concern regarding possible exposure to sexually transmitted diseases. During your pelvic examination, a single, indurated, nontender ulcer is noted on the vulva. Venereal Disease Research Laboratory (VDRL) and fluorescent treponemal antibody (FTA) tests are positive. Without treatment, the next stage of this disease is clinically characterized by which of the following?

a. Optic nerve atrophy and generalized paresis
b. Tabes dorsalis
c. Gummas
d. Macular rash over the hands and feet
e. Aortic aneurysm

8-18. You are seeing a healthy 26-year-old woman for a routine health visit. She mentions that she and her husband are thinking about starting a family soon. She has never been pregnant before. Which of the following interventions, if done prior to pregnancy, has been shown to have a clear beneficial outcome for this woman and her potential child?

a. Blood typing and antibody testing
b. Screening for HIV
c. Screening for *Chlamydia*
d. Screening for asymptomatic bacteriuria
e. Prescribing 0.4 to 0.8 mg of folic acid daily

8-19. A 41-year-old man underwent a successful living related kidney transplantation 1 year previously with good results. Preoperatively, he was noted to have an elevated calcium level; posttransplantation, he continues to have elevated calcium levels and associated symptoms. Which of the following is the most appropriate next step in management?

a. ^{99m}Tc sestamibi scanning
b. Ultrasound of the neck
c. CT scan of the neck and mediastinum
d. Total parathyroidectomy with autotransplantation of a portion of a gland into the forearm
e. Measurement of urinary calcium levels

8-20. A 78-year-old woman with mild Alzheimer disease falls at home and suffers a left hip fracture. She is admitted to the hospital and undergoes a left total hip replacement. Postoperatively she is given D5W and treated with meperidine for pain, diphenhydramine for sleep, and given prophylactic ranitidine. On the second postoperative day, she pulls out her Foley catheter and her IV. On examination blood pressure is 150/90, pulse rate is 80, and temperature 36.7°C (98°F). Oxygen saturation on room air is 92%. She is markedly confused and appears agitated. She has no focal neurologic findings. Laboratory testing reveals WBC = 7500, hemoglobin = 10.2, Na = 132, potassium = 3.2, BUN = 6, creatinine = 0.9. CXR, ECG, and liver tests are normal. What is the next best step in her management?

a. Order CT scan of the brain.
b. Order ventilation perfusion lung scan.
c. Obtain blood cultures and begin broad-spectrum antibiotics.
d. Restrain the patient and order lorazepam for agitation.
e. Remove Foley catheter, change fluids to NS with KCL, and discontinue meperidine, diphenhydramine, and ranitidine.

8-21. A middle-aged woman presents with a variety of cognitive and somatic symptoms, fatigue, and memory loss. She denies feeling sad, but her family physician is aware of this patient's lifelong inability to identify and express feelings. He suspects she is depressed. Which of the following results is most likely to confirm a diagnosis of depression?

a. Reduced metabolic activity and blood flow in both frontal lobes on PET scan
b. Diffuse cortical atrophy on CAT scan
c. Atrophy of the caudate on MRI
d. Prolonged REM sleep latency in a sleep study
e. Subcortical infarcts on MRI

8-22. A 37-year-old man has an MRI performed by his primary care doctor because of a long history of headaches. It is notable only for the finding of a type 1 Chiari malformation. He is sent to a neurologist for further evaluation. A type 1 Chiari malformation usually becomes symptomatic as which of the following in adults?

a. Epilepsy
b. Hydrocephalus
c. Ataxia
d. Dementia
e. Psychosis

Questions 23 to 24

8-23. An off-Broadway actor consistently bores his friends and acquaintances by talking incessantly about his exceptional talent and his success on the stage. He does not seem to realize that other people do not share his high opinion of his acting talent and are not interested in his monologues. When a director criticizes the way he delivers his lines during rehearsal, the actor goes into a rage and accuses the director of trying to jeopardize his career out of jealousy. Which personality disorder represents the most likely diagnosis?

a. Histrionic
b. Narcissistic
c. Borderline
d. Paranoid
e. Antisocial

8-24. The patient in the vignette above seeks out a psychiatrist because, he says, "It is depressing when no one understands your talent." Which of the following treatments would be most appropriate?

a. Medication with an SSRI
b. Medication with a tricyclic antidepressant
c. Group psychotherapy with patients from a wide range of other diagnoses
d. Psychoanalysis
e. Psychodynamic psychotherapy

8-25. A 42-year-old man is undergoing chemotherapy after resection of a cecal adenocarcinoma with positive lymph nodes. You are asked to see him regarding a potential surgical complication. Which of the following potentially operable complications is a common occurrence among patients receiving systemic chemotherapy?

a. Acute cholecystitis
b. Perirectal abscess
c. Appendicitis
d. Incarcerated femoral hernia
e. Diverticulitis

8-26. A 4-year-old boy is brought to the physician by his parents because he experiences episodes of waking in the middle of the night and screaming. The parents state that when they get to the boy's room during one of these episodes, they find him in his bed, thrashing wildly, his eyes wide open. He pushes them away when they try to comfort him. After 2 minutes, the boy suddenly falls asleep, and the next day he has no memory of the episode. Which of the following medications should be the first choice to treat this disorder?

a. Haloperidol
b. Diazepam
c. Methylphenidate
d. Amitriptyline
e. Valproic acid

8-27. A 34-year-old G1P1 who delivered her first baby 5 weeks ago calls your office and asks to speak with you. She tells you that she is feeling very overwhelmed and anxious. She feels that she cannot do anything right and feels sad throughout the day. She tells you that she finds herself crying all the time and is unable to sleep at night. Which of the following is the most likely diagnosis?

a. Postpartum depression
b. Maternity blues
c. Postpartum psychosis
d. Bipolar disease
e. Postpartum blues

8-28. You are taking care of a 32-year-old woman with mild hypertension, arthritis, and depression. She presents to you complaining of a sore throat without cough or congestion. You diagnose her with pharyngitis and begin treatment. She then has an acute onset of hematuria, and comes to your office for evaluation. Which of the following medications used to treat pharyngitis is the most likely cause?

a. Ibuprofen
b. Penicillin
c. Azithromycin
d. Erythromycin
e. Ciprofloxacin

8-29. A 13-year-old boy has a 3-day history of low-grade fever, symptoms of upper respiratory infection, and a sore throat. A few hours before his presentation to the emergency room, he has an abrupt onset of high fever, difficulty swallowing, and poor handling of his secretions. He indicates that he has a marked worsening in the severity of his sore throat. His pharynx has a fluctuant bulge in the posterior wall. A soft tissue radiograph of his neck is shown. Which of the following is the most appropriate initial therapy for this patient?

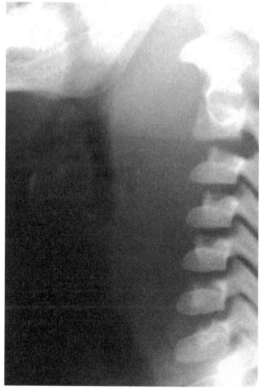

(Used with permission from Susan John, MD.)

a. Narcotic analgesics
b. Trial of oral penicillin V
c. Surgical consultation for incision and drainage under general anesthesia
d. Rapid streptococcal screen
e. Monospot test

8-30. A thorough evaluation reveals that a 69-year-old patient has a symptomatic 90% stenosis of the right internal carotid artery at the bifurcation. Which of the following management options is most likely to prevent a future stroke?

a. Warfarin
b. Carotid artery angioplasty
c. Carotid endarterectomy
d. Extracranial-intracranial bypass
e. Aspirin

8-31. A 25-year-old man fell off his surfboard and landed on rocks. He was pulled from the water by lifeguards and brought to the ED in full cervical and spinal immobilization. He is alert and oriented to person, place, and time. He is complaining of weakness in all of his extremities. His temperature is 98.4°F, BP is 85/50 mm Hg, HR is 60 beats per minute, RR is 20 breaths per minute, and oxygen saturation is 98% on room air. On examination, he has no external signs of head injury. His heart is bradycardic without murmurs. The lungs are clear to auscultation and the abdomen is soft and nontender. He has grossly normal peripheral sensation, but no motor strength in all four extremities. Which of the following is the most likely diagnosis?

a. Hypovolemic shock
b. Neurogenic shock
c. Cardiogenic shock
d. Anaphylactic shock
e. Septic shock

8-32. You are caring for a 9-year-old whose mother brought him in for evaluation of his sore throat. He has been ill for 24 hours. In addition to the sore throat, he has a fever, but no cough. On physical examination, his temperature is 101°F, tender anterior cervical adenopathy and tonsillar exudate. Which of the following is the next best step in his care?

a. Reassurance and observation for a few more days
b. Perform a rapid streptococcal screening test
c. Perform a throat culture
d. Treat with penicillin
e. Treat with steroids

8-33. A patient who has had angina as well as claudication reports feeling light-headed on exertion, especially when lifting and working with his arms. The subclavian steal syndrome is associated with which of the following hemodynamic abnormalities?

a. Antegrade flow through a vertebral artery
b. Venous congestion of the upper extremities
c. Occlusion of the carotid artery
d. Occlusion of the vertebral artery
e. Occlusion of the subclavian artery

8-34. A 40-year-old female presents to your office regarding a breast lump she found on self-examination 2 weeks ago. The patient does not regularly examine her breasts. Her last clinical breast examination was 2 years ago; mammogram 9 months ago was normal with recommendation for follow-up mammogram in 1 year. She has no family members with breast cancer. Her father had colon cancer diagnosed 10 years ago. She takes no medications regularly. On examination, she has a well-localized nontender nodule in the left breast at 2 o'clock. It is approximately 1.5 cm in diameter with irregular borders. Diagnostic breast imaging includes a negative mammogram and a sonogram that reveals a solid area in the left breast at the site of the palpable abnormality. Which of the following is the most appropriate next step?

a. Reassure your patient and follow-up in 6 months.
b. Refer the patient for needle biopsy.
c. Tell the patient to discontinue caffeine and wear a supportive bra.
d. Schedule a CT scan of the thorax.
e. Start the patient on NSAIDs and vitamin E.

8-35. A 29-year-old G1P0 presents to the obstetrician's office at 41 weeks gestation. On physical examination, her cervix is 1 centimeter dilated, 0% effaced, firm, and posterior in position. The vertex is presenting at −3 station. Which of the following is the best next step in the management of this patient?

a. Send the patient to the hospital for induction of labor since she has a favorable Bishop score.
b. Teach the patient to measure fetal kick counts and deliver her if at any time there are less than 20 perceived fetal movements in 3 hours.
c. Order BPP testing for the same or next day.
d. Schedule the patient for induction of labor at 43 weeks gestation.
e. Schedule cesarean delivery for the following day since it is unlikely that the patient will go into labor.

8-36. A 22-year-old student is in therapy because he has a long history of chaotic interpersonal relationships, episodes of psychosis, and multiple hospitalizations. He has attempted suicide three times, mostly precipitated by his feeling overwhelmed in some social setting. One session, he comes to his therapist greatly upset and anxious because he forgot to study some material that will be on an upcoming examination. The therapist reminds the patient that he has done well on previous examinations and suggests that they spend the session devising a study plan for the time the patient has left before the test. Such an intervention is commonly used in which of the following therapies?

a. Psychoanalysis
b. Object relation psychotherapy
c. Cognitive-behavioral therapy
d. Supportive psychotherapy
e. Interpersonal psychotherapy

8-37. A 24-year-old G0 presents to your office complaining of vulvar discomfort. More specifically, she has been experiencing intense burning and pain with intercourse. The discomfort occurs at the vaginal introitus primarily with penile insertion into the vagina. The patient also experiences the same pain with tampon insertion and when the speculum is inserted during a gynecologic examination. The problem has become so severe that she can no longer have sex, which is causing problems in her marriage. She is otherwise healthy and denies any medical problems. She is experiencing regular menses and denies any dysmenorrhea. On physical examination, the region of the vulva around the vaginal vestibule has several punctate, erythematous areas of epithelium measuring 3 to 8 mm in diameter. Most of the lesions are located on the skin between the two Bartholin glands. Each inflamed lesion is tender to touch with a cotton swab. Which of the following is the most likely diagnosis?

a. Vulvar vestibulitis
b. Atrophic vaginitis
c. Contact dermatitis
d. Lichen sclerosus
e. Vulvar intraepithelial neoplasia

8-38. A 56-year-old right-handed woman presents to the emergency room with a sudden-onset, severe, left-sided headache. The pain began when she stood up from her couch while watching TV. A head CT is normal. Which of the following is the most appropriate next step in management of this patient?

a. Begin intravenous heparin
b. Perform a lumbar puncture
c. Obtain a brain MRI
d. Obtain a cerebral angiogram
e. Give the patient a prescription for zolmitriptan and send her home

8-39. One of your patients with polycystic ovarian syndrome presents to the emergency room complaining of prolonged, heavy vaginal bleeding. She is 26 years old and has never been pregnant. She was taking birth control pills to regulate her periods until 4 months ago. She stopped taking them because she and her spouse want to try to get pregnant. She thought she might be pregnant because she had not had a period since her last one on the birth control pills 4 months ago. She started having vaginal bleeding 8 days ago. She has been doubling up on superabsorbant sanitary napkins 5 to 6 times daily since the bleeding began. On arrival at the emergency room, the patient has a supine blood pressure of 102/64 mm Hg with a pulse of 96 beats per minute. Upon standing, the patient feels light-headed. Her standing blood pressure is 108/66 mm Hg with a pulse of 126 beats per minute. While you wait for lab work to come back, you order intravenous hydration. After 2 hours, the patient is no longer orthostatic. Her pregnancy test comes back negative, and her Hct is 31%. She continues to have heavy bleeding. Which of the following is the best next step in the management of this patient?

a. Perform a dilation and curettage.
b. Administer a blood transfusion to treat her severe anemia.
c. Send her home with a prescription for iron therapy.
d. Administer high-dose estrogen therapy.
e. Administer antiprostaglandins.

Questions 40 to 43

For each clinical scenario below, select the most likely diagnosis. Each lettered option may be used once, more than once, or not at all.

a. Bronchopulmonary dysplasia
b. Respiratory distress syndrome (hyaline membrane disease)
c. Pulmonary interstitial emphysema
d. Bronchiolitis
e. Primary pulmonary hypoplasia
f. Pneumothorax
g. Asthma
h. Meconium aspiration
i. Phrenic nerve paralysis
j. Bacterial pneumonia

8-40. A large-for-gestation-age term infant is delivered via scheduled cesarean section develops, at 15 minutes of age, tachypnea, grunting, flaring, and retractions. The child does not move his left arm well, but you find no clavicular fracture. A chest radiograph shows the left diaphragm to be markedly higher than the right.

8-41. A postterm infant is born at home after a prolonged and difficult labor. The maternal grandmother brings the infant to the hospital at 1 hour of life because of fast breathing. Grandmother notes that the child seemed well for a while, but then developed increased work of breathing. Physical examination reveals an infant in moderate respiratory distress with diminished breath sounds on the left. Chest radiograph reveals the heart to be pushed to the right side and loss of lung markings in the left lung field.

8-42. An infant of uncertain but seemingly term dates is born via emergent cesarean section for nonreassuring heart tones; the obstetrician has noted little or no amniotic fluid. The infant is small, has abnormally shaped limbs, and an unusual facies. The child has immediate respiratory distress. A chest radiograph reveals a poorly developed chest with little lung tissue.

8-43. A preterm infant is now 7 weeks old. She was intubated for 2 weeks and was weaned off oxygen at 3 weeks of age. You are about to leave your office for Thanksgiving holiday when the emergency room calls to tell you she has new hypoxia, respiratory distress, wheezes, and runny nose. A chest radiograph reveals patchy infiltrates and hyperexpansion in both lung fields. The newborn's 2-year-old sibling has an upper respiratory infection.

Questions 44 to 46

For each of the clinical situations below, select the most likely diagnosis. Each lettered option may be used once, more than once, or not at all.

a. Tuberculosis
b. Primary lung tumor
c. Pulmonary embolus
d. Metastatic lung cancer
e. Asbestosis
f. Histoplasmosis
g. Idiopathic pulmonary fibrosis

8-44. A 32-year-old male has cough with yellow, blood-tinged sputum. He also has a history of night sweats and a 10-lb weight loss. The patient was born in India. On physical examination there is dullness to percussion above both clavicles. Chest x-ray shows bilateral upper lobe infiltrates with cavity formation.

8-45. A 55-year-old woman who is a heavy cigarette smoker complains of cough with small amounts of bright red blood. She has also noted loss of appetite and a 12-lb weight loss. A 3-cm pulmonary nodule with shaggy margins is seen on chest x-ray.

8-46. A 65-year-old who is retiring from work as a plumber has complained of a dry cough. He has also had some shortness of breath on walking. On physical examination there are bilateral crackling rales at both lung bases. Bilateral clubbing is also noted. On chest x-ray, bilateral linear infiltrates are seen at the lung bases. Pleural scarring is noted on CT scan.

Block 1

Answers

1-1. The answer is e. *(Tintinalli, pp 352-353.)* Thrombolytic therapy (clot-busters) can be administered to patients having an acute ST-elevation MI that is within 6 to 12 hours from symptom onset. Contraindications to fibrinolytic therapy are those that increase the risk of hemorrhage. The most catastrophic complication is intracranial hemorrhage. Absolute contraindications include:

- Previous hemorrhagic stroke
- Known intracranial neoplasm
- Active internal bleeding (excluding menses)
- Suspected aortic dissection or pericarditis

(a) SBP > 180 mm Hg is a relative contraindication. However, if thrombolytics are going to be administered and the patient's SBP is > 180 mm Hg, antihypertensive medication can be administered to lower the SBP to below 180 mm Hg. (b) Anticoagulation is a relative contraindication. Many patients who suffer from an ST-elevation MI are on aspirin and other antiplatelet and anticoagulant therapies. (c) Major surgery less than 3 weeks prior to administration of thrombolytics is a relative contraindication. (d) Active peptic ulcer disease is a relative contraindication.

1-2. The answer is c. *(Townsend, p 713.)* Hyperacute rejection occurs within minutes after transplantation and is mediated primarily by preformed antibody. It usually occurs during surgery after the clamps are released from the vascular anastomosis and the recipient's antibodies are exposed to the donor's passenger lymphocytes and kidney tissue. Typically, the kidney will become swollen and bluish. Intraoperative biopsies of the transplanted kidney should be performed to evaluate for signs of hyperacute rejection such as extensive intravascular deposits of fibrin and platelets and intraglomerular accumulation of polymorphonuclear leukocytes, fibrin, platelets, and red blood cells. The intravascular coagulation rarely results in a systemic coagulopathy. Careful cross-matching can test for cytotoxic antibodies and prevent hyperacute rejections. Hyperacute rejection is refractory to immunosuppressive or anticoagulant therapy and inevitably leads to rapid destruction of the transplanted kidney.

1-3. The answer is b. (*Jacobson, pp 85-91.*) The essential features of obsessive-compulsive disorder are obsessions (recurrent and persistent thoughts that are experienced as intrusive and inappropriate and that cause anxiety) and compulsions (repetitive behaviors that the person feels driven to perform). In this disorder, the patient's symptoms are ego-dystonic to him or her, unlike the person with an obsessive-compulsive personality disorder. Patients with attention-deficit hyperactivity disorder have problems with inattention, hyperactivity, and/or impulsivity. Patients with separation anxiety disorder worry about losing or harming major attachment figures and become anxious when separation from home or those major figures is anticipated. Patients with brief psychotic disorder show evidence of either delusions or hallucinations for a short period of time, usually after exposure to some external stressor.

1-4. The answer is c. (*Cunningham, pp 867-873.*) The patient is in preterm labor, because she has a dilated and effaced cervix in the presence of regular uterine contractions. Therefore, treatment is aimed at delaying delivery to allow continued fetal growth and maturity. The administration of tocolytic therapy to treat the preterm contractions is indicated. In addition, from 24 to 34 weeks, management also includes the administration of steroids, such as betamethasone, to promote fetal lung maturity. Respiratory distress syndrome is a sequela of preterm neonates and occurs less often in infants given betamethasone in utero. If delivery seems likely, intravenous antibiotics are administered to prevent possible neonatal sepsis. If the patient's contractions subside and there is no evidence of infection, then the antibiotics can be discontinued. It is advantageous to obtain a neonatology consult on any patient who appears to be in preterm labor so the parents know what to expect if they give birth to preterm infants. There is no need to prepare for a cesarean section in this patient. Attempts are made to stop the labor first. If the patient continues to progress, then a vaginal delivery is preferred since the twins do not have a malpresentation.

1-5. The answer is b. (*Ropper, pp 16-18.*) Calcified masses appear hyperdense without contrast enhancement, whereas highly vascular lesions may appear dense on CT scanning after the patient has received intravenous contrast material. Tumors, granulomas, and other intracranial lesions enhance because of a breakdown in the blood—brain barrier. More cystic lesions may exhibit enhancement limited to the periphery of the cyst.

1-6 to 1-10. The answers are 6-d, 7-a, 8-b, 9-e, 10-c. *(Greenfield, pp 1466-1468.)* The Argyll Robertson pupil (a pupil that constricts with accommodation but not in response to light) is characteristic of central nervous system syphilis and is associated with vascular system manifestations of that disease. *Treponema pallidum* invades the vasa vasorum and causes an obliterative endarteritis and necrosis. The resulting aortitis gradually weakens the aortic wall and predisposes it to aneurysm formation. Once an aneurysm has formed, the prognosis is grave. Massive isolated tricuspid regurgitation produces a markedly elevated venous pressure, usually manifested by a severely engorged (often pulsating) liver. If the venous pressure is sufficiently elevated, exophthalmos may result. Tricuspid regurgitation of rheumatic origin is almost never an isolated lesion, and the major symptoms of patients who have rheumatic heart disease are usually attributable to concurrent left heart lesions. Bacterial endocarditis from intravenous drug abuse is becoming an increasingly important cause of isolated tricuspid regurgitation. A Quincke pulse, which consists of alternate flushing and paling of the skin or nail beds, is associated with aortic regurgitation. Other characteristic features of the peripheral pulse in aortic regurgitation include the waterhammer pulse (Corrigan pulse, caused by a rapid systolic upstroke) and pulsus bisferiens, which describes a double systolic hump in the pulse contour. The finding of a wide pulse pressure provides an additional diagnostic clue to aortic regurgitation. Myocarditis, aortitis, and pericarditis have all been described in association with Reiter syndrome; the original description included conjunctivitis, urethritis, and arthralgias. Although its cause is unknown, Reiter syndrome is associated with HLA-B27 antigen, as are aortic regurgitation, pericarditis, and ankylosing spondylitis. Short stature, webbed neck, low-set ears, and epicanthal folds are the classic features of patients who have Turner syndrome. Persons affected by the syndrome, which is commonly linked with aortic coarctation, are genotypically XO. However, females and males have been described with normal sex chromosome constitutions (XX, XY) but with the phenotypic abnormalities of Turner syndrome. Additional cardiac lesions associated with Turner syndrome include septal defects, valvular stenosis, and anomalies of the great vessels.

1-11. The answer is c. *(Fauci, pp 908-914, 2621-2624.)* This previously healthy male has developed acute bacterial meningitis as evident by meningeal irritation with a positive Brudzinski sign, and a CSF profile typical for bacterial meningitis (elevated white blood cell count, high percentage of polymorphonuclear leukocytes, elevated protein, and low glucose). The patient likely has concomitant pneumonia. This combination suggests pneumococcal infection, and the CSF Gram stain confirms *S pneumoniae* as the etiologic agent. Because of the potential for beta-lactam resistance, the recommendation for therapy prior to availability of susceptibility data is ceftriaxone and vancomycin. Though herpes simplex is a common problem in young healthy patients, the clinical picture and CSF profile are not consistent with this infection. The CSF in herpes simplex encephalitis shows a lymphocytic predominance and normal glucose. *Listeria monocytogenes* meningitis is a concern in immunocompromised and elderly patients. Gram stain would show gram-positive rods. *Neisseria meningitidis* is the second commonest cause of bacterial meningitis but rarely causes pneumonia (the portal of entry is the nasopharynx). Gram stain of meningococci would show gram-negative diplococci. Because the patient has no papilledema and no focal neurologic findings, treatment should not be delayed to obtain an MRI scan.

1-12. The answer is a. (*Hay, pp 192-194. Kliegman, pp 124-125. McMillan, pp 648-650. Rudolph, pp 501-503.*) The adolescent who has attempted suicide should be hospitalized so that a complete medical, psychological, and social evaluation can be performed and an appropriate treatment plan developed. Hospitalization also emphasizes the seriousness of the adolescent's action to her and to her family and the importance of cooperation in carrying out the recommendations for ongoing future therapy. The treatment plan may include continued counseling or supportive therapy with a pediatrician, outpatient psychotherapy with a psychiatrist or other mental health worker, or family therapy.

1-13. The answer is b. (*Cunningham, pp 627-628.*) With velamentous insertion of the cord, the umbilical vessels separate in the membranes at a distance from the placental margin, which they reach surrounded only by amnion. It occurs in about 1% of singleton gestations but is quite common in multiple pregnancies. Fetal malformations are more common with velamentous insertion of the umbilical cord. When fetal vessels cross the internal os (vasa previa), rupture of membranes may be accompanied by rupture of a fetal vessel, leading to fetal exsanguination. Vasa previa does not increase the risk for placenta accreta or amniotic fluid embolism. An increased risk of premature rupture of membranes and of torsion of the umbilical cord has not been described in association with velamentous insertion of the cord.

1-14. The answer is e. (*Roberts and Hedges, pp 19-24.*) Patients frequently present to the ED with agitation. It is important to discern what is causing their agitation; the range of etiologies is expansive, from ethanol intoxication to intracerebral bleeding. The approach to the emergency patient always begins with the **ABCs (airway, breathing, and circulation)**. In addition, the **vital signs** must be obtained early in a patient's assessment in order **to reveal potentially life-threatening conditions**. The patient in the vignette presents with agitation and tachycardia. Although it is tempting to attribute his agitation to his untreated schizophrenia, doing this without investigating medical causes of agitation can be disastrous. Finding out that the patient's temperature is 103.1°F, for instance, will lead you down a different clinical path than if his temperature is 98°F. This patient was ultimately diagnosed with meningitis.

(**a**) Administering a medication to control agitation or psychotic behavior is appropriate even when there are coexistent medical problems. Patients that are too agitated cannot be properly examined. However, it is critical to rule out potential life threats that may be causing the agitation. (**b**) A psychiatry consultation should be obtained once life-threatening conditions are excluded or in the case of the patient above, when he is stable and communicative as an inpatient. (**c and d**) A head CT and blood work will need to be obtained in this patient; however, all of the vital signs should be obtained first.

1-15. The answer is b. (*South-Paul, pp 310-328.*) The first priority when evaluating abdominal pain is to determine whether the pain is acute or chronic. Sudden and/or severe onset of pain should lead the clinician toward an emergent evaluation. Right lower quadrant pain is suspicious for an acute appendicitis, but by itself is not specific enough to warrant an emergent workup. A "gnawing" sensation is often described with ulcer disease, while pain that worsens after eating is associated with many conditions—pancreatitis, gallbladder disease, or even reflux. In the absence of hemodynamic instability, those causes are less likely to warrant emergent workup. Emesis with pain is not enough, by itself, to warrant emergent workup.

1-16. The answer is b. (*Kaplan, pp 830-832.*) Pancreatic carcinoma should always be considered in depressed middle-aged patients. It presents with weight loss, abdominal pain, apathy, decreased energy, lethargy, anhedonia, and depression. An elevated amylase can sometimes be found in laboratory testing. The other disorders listed do not present in this manner.

1-17. The answer is b. (*Brunicardi, p 1636.*) This T1-weighted sagittal MRI scan reveals a dumbbell-shaped homogeneous mass involving the sella turcica and the suprasellar region. This lesion is most consistent with a pituitary adenoma, a benign tumor arising from the adenohypophysis. Pituitary adenomas are the most common sellar lesion and constitute 10% to 15% of all intracranial neoplasms. Macroadenomas are greater than 1 cm in size and microadenomas less than 1 cm. Pituitary adenomas may be functional, resulting in endocrinopathies from excessive hormone secretion, such as prolactin (amenorrhea or galactorrhea), growth hormone (gigantism or acromegaly), or adrenocorticotrophic hormone (ACTH) (Cushing syndrome). The tumor pictured is a macroadenoma; these larger tumors may cause symptoms secondary to mass effect; for example, a bitemporal visual field defect can result from compression of the optic chiasm. This tumor's dumbbell shape results from impingement on the adenoma by the diaphragm of the sella turcica. The suprasellar extension seen here makes a frontal craniotomy rather than the more commonly utilized transsphenoidal approach more appropriate.

1-18. The answer is c. (*Ropper, pp 757-758.*) Something has abruptly caused increasing intracranial pressure in this young man after his head trauma. Consequently, he is at risk for herniation of the brain transfalcially (across the falx cerebri) or transtentorially (across the tentorium cerebelli). The head trauma produced an intracranial lesion, which is expanding very rapidly. The slowing of his pulse and increase in his blood pressure are due to the Cushing effect of a rapidly expanding intracranial mass. The history is typical for that of an epidural hematoma.

1-19. The answer is e. (*Brunicardi, pp 1436-1437.*) Osteitis fibrosa cystica is a condition associated with hyperparathyroidism that is characterized by severe demineralization with subperiosteal bone resorption (most prominent in the middle phalanx of the second and third fingers), bone cysts, and tufting of the distal phalanges on hand films. These specific bone findings would not be present in sarcoidosis, Paget disease, or metastatic carcinoma. Vitamin D deficiency can lead to osteitis fibrosa cystica but it would also be associated with hypocalcemia, not hypercalcemia.

1-20. The answer is e. (*Kaplan, p 28.*) The term *stranger anxiety* refers to manifestations of discomfort and distress on the part of the infant when he or she is approached by a stranger. Although it does not necessarily appear every time the child meets a stranger, and although some children seem to be more prone than others to such reactions, stranger anxiety is considered a normal, transient phenomenon. It manifests at about 8 months of age, when the child starts differentiating between familiar and unfamiliar adults.

1-21. The answer is c. (*Mengel, pp 60-66.*) In dementia, the level of consciousness is not clouded, but disorientation may occur later in the illness. Hypertension and diabetes may be seen with both delirium and dementia. The inability to complete serial sevens (count backward from 100 by 7s) may be related to educational level. Although his symptoms have appeared recently, it is often difficult to pinpoint the exact onset of dementia. Delirium is seen as being more abrupt in onset.

1-22. The answer is c. (*Rakel, pp 5-10.*) While all of the medications listed have antiemetic properties, the patient described has gastroparesis, likely as a result of her longstanding diabetes. Metoclopramide can improve gastric motility and help her symptoms more than the other antiemetics listed.

1-23. The answer is d. (*Rosen, pp 1176-1185.*) The **classic triad** of a **ruptured abdominal aortic aneurysm (AAA)** is **pain, hypotension**, and a **pulsatile abdominal mass.** Sometimes patients have only one or two of the components and occasionally may have none. Most patients who are diagnosed with AAA are asymptomatic. However, rupture is often the first manifestation of an AAA. Most patients with a ruptured AAA experience pain in the abdomen, back, or flank. It is usually acute in onset and severe. Approximately 20% of the time, patients present to the ED with syncope. Patients with a ruptured AAA are unstable until their aorta is cross clamped in the OR. Therefore, any **hemodynamically unstable** patient with a diagnosed or strongly suspected AAA should be **taken immediately to the OR.**
(a) A CT scan is excellent for diagnosing an AAA in stable patients. (b) Angiography has no role in the emergent evaluation of a patient suspected of a ruptured AAA. (c) An abdominal radiograph can aid in the diagnosis of an AAA. However, when there is high clinical suspicion and the patient is hemodynamically unstable, the patient should be brought to the OR. (e) The patient is not complaining of chest pain and his ECG is not consistent with an acute coronary event. Therefore, cardiac catheterization is not required.

1-24. The answer is c. (*Rock, pp 1084-1089.*) The patient most likely has a ureteral injury at the location of the left uterine artery. A noninvasive renal ultrasound is fast, inexpensive, and accurate way to make the diagnosis. Intravenous pyelograms although used in the past are outdated tests and have been replaced by use of computed tomography (CT). A CT scan with contrast gives excellent information on the integrity and function of the renal collecting system; however, when the serum creatinine is elevated, intravenous contrast can cause significant renal damage and is contraindicated in those circumstances. A chest x-ray would not be helpful in making the diagnosis. Intravenous antibiotics are not indicated at this time since there is not clear evidence of an infection (normal white blood cell count). A ureteral injury itself will cause a temperature elevation. The patient has a normal drop in hemoglobin for the surgical blood loss and does not have signs of hemodynamic instability to warrant a blood transfusion at this time.

1-25. The answer is e. *(Hay, pp 708-711, 764-765. Kliegman, pp 2440-2441, 2513-2521. McMillan, pp 924-933, 2679-2680. Rudolph, pp 900-904, 2169.)* Unsuspected bacteremia caused by *H influenzae* type B (now rare), *Neisseria meningitidis*, or *S pneumoniae* (decreasing in frequency secondary to vaccination) should be considered before prescribing treatment for otitis media in a young, febrile, toxic-appearing infant. In this situation, blood culture should be performed before antibiotic therapy is initiated, and examination of the CSF is indicated if meningitis is suspected.

The classic signs of meningitis are found with increasing reliability in children older than 6 months. Nevertheless, a febrile, irritable, inconsolable infant with an altered state of alertness deserves a lumbar puncture even in the absence of meningeal signs. A petechial rash, characteristically associated with meningococcal infection, has been known to occur with other bacterial infections as well. Organisms may be identified on smear of these lesions.

A fever accompanied by inability to flex rather than rotate the neck immediately suggests meningitis (a sign more reliable in children older than 12 to 18 months of age). An indolent clinical course does not rule out bacterial meningitis. A lumbar puncture is of prime diagnostic importance in determining the presence of bacterial meningitis, which requires immediate antibiotic therapy. A delay in treatment can lead to complications such as cerebrovascular thrombosis, obstructive hydrocephalus, cerebritis with seizures or acute increased intracranial pressure, coma, or death. A missed diagnosis of meningitis is one of the most common reasons for civil litigation involving a pediatrician. In the described patient, lumbar puncture is warranted because of the change in his clinical status.

1-26. The answer is e. *(Fauci, pp 115-117, 2154.)* Shoulder pain may be caused by inflammation of tendons or muscles in the shoulder girdle, intra-articular problems at the glenohumeral joint, or referred pain from a cervical radiculopathy. Posterior shoulder pain and a normal shoulder examination are clues to the correct diagnosis in this patient. The pain of cervical radiculopathy is often severe and worse at night. Extension of pain into the arm may occur, but this also occurs with other etiologies of shoulder pain. Shoulder pain is common, particularly in the elderly. Subdeltoid bursitis causes exquisite local tenderness. Rotator cuff tendonitis is frequently associated with pain on active but not passive movement of the joint. Weakness of the arm suggests rotator cuff tear. In adhesive capsulitis, range of motion is restricted. Crepitance on manipulation of the shoulder suggests osteoarthritis of the glenohumoral joint.

1-27. The answer is a. (*Fauci, pp 2175-2177.*) The patient's multiple tender points, associated sleep disturbance and lack of joint or muscle findings make fibromyalgia a likely diagnosis. Patients with fibromyalgia often report dropping things due to pain and weakness, but objective muscle weakness is not present on examination. The diagnosis hinges on the presence of multiple tender points in the absence of any other disease likely to cause musculoskeletal symptoms. CBC and ESR are characteristically normal. Cognitive behavioral therapy and graded aerobic exercise programs have been demonstrated to relieve symptoms. Tricyclic antidepressants may help restore sleep. Aspirin, other anti-inflammatory drugs (including corticosteroids), and DMARDs (such as methotrexate or hydroxychloroquine) are not helpful. Neither are simple stretching/flexibility exercises. Of note, rheumatoid factor and antinuclear antibodies occur in a small number of normal individuals. They are more frequent in women and increase in frequency with age. It is not uncommon for an individual with fibromyalgia and an incidentally positive RF or ANA to be misdiagnosed as having collagen vascular disease. Therefore, it is necessary to be careful to separate subjective tenderness on examination from objective musculoskeletal findings and to assiduously search for other criteria before diagnosing RA, SLE, or other collagen vascular disease.

1-28. The answer is d. (*Ropper, pp 58, 85.*) Young adults who have self-administered MPTP in an effort to achieve an opiate high have developed progressive damage to the substantia nigra. The neurologic syndrome that results from this damage is indistinguishable from Parkinson disease, except that it evolves over weeks or months rather than years. Affected persons exhibit rigidity, tremor, and bradykinesia. That a toxin can produce a syndrome indistinguishable from Parkinson disease has increased speculation that some—perhaps many—persons with Parkinson disease have had environmental exposure to a toxin that produced degeneration of the substantia nigra.

I-29. The answer is a. *(Townsend, pp 489-493.)* Acute signs of airway distress (stridor, hoarseness, dysphonia), visceral injury (subcutaneous air, hemoptysis, dysphagia), hemorrhage (expanding hematoma, unchecked external bleeding), and neurologic symptoms referable to carotid injury (stroke or altered mental status) or lower cranial nerve or brachial plexus injury requires formal neck exploration. Pneumothorax would mandate a chest tube; the necessity for exploration would depend on clinical judgment and institutional policy. Additionally, all hemodynamically unstable patients with a penetrating neck wound should be explored, while management of asymptomatic, stable patients with neck injuries that penetrate the platysma is more controversial. In the past, treatment of asymptomatic, stable patients with zone II (between the lower border of the cricoid cartilage to the angle of the mandible) injuries was mandatory operative exploration. However, proponents for selective management of these patients argue that there is a high rate of negative explorations of the neck (40%-60%) and that serious injuries can be overlooked despite operative exploration. Furthermore, studies have demonstrated similar incidences of overall mortality with either selective or mandatory exploration. Stable patients with zone III (between the angle of the mandible and the skull), zone I (between the sternal notch and the lower border of the cricoid cartilage), or multiple neck wounds, should undergo initial angiography irrespective of the ultimate treatment plan. For zone II injuries, algorithms exist for nonoperative management of asymptomatic patients that employ observation alone or combinations of vascular and aerodigestive contrast studies and endoscopy.

I-30. The answer is a. *(Kaplan, pp 1056-1058.)* Lithium has been proven effective when added to an antidepressant in the treatment of refractory depression. More than one mechanism of action is probably involved, although lithium's ability to increase the presynaptic release of serotonin is the best understood. Other augmentation strategies include the use of thyroid hormones, stimulants, estrogens, and light therapy. The combination of two SSRIs (in this case, fluoxetine and sertraline) or of an MAOI and an SSRI is not recommended because of the risk of precipitating a serotonin syndrome.

I-31. The answer is d. *(ACIP, 2007a.)* Of the vaccines listed, only the pneumococcal polysaccharide vaccine is indicated for people who have chronic pulmonary disease. She should receive a one-time administration, since she is over the age of 65. Had she received her initial shot before the age of 65, she would require a one-time "booster" shot, 5 years after the initial one. People born before 1957 do not need to be vaccinated with an

MMR, as they are considered immune. People born before 1980 are considered immune to varicella. The Tdap vaccine is only indicated for those under the age of 65, and intranasal influenza should only be used in healthy adults under the age of 50.

I-32. The answer is b. (*Hay, pp 413, 1272. Kliegman, pp 2756-2758. McMillan, pp 847, 863, 1382-1383. Rudolph, pp 1153-1154, 1233-1234.*) Scabies is caused by the mite *Sarcoptes scabiei var. hominis.* Most older children and adults present with intensely pruritic and threadlike burrows in the interdigital areas, groin, elbows, and ankles; the palms, soles, face, and head are spared. Infants, however, usually present with bullae and pustules, and the areas spared in adults are often involved in infants. The clinical manifestations closely resemble those of atopic dermatitis. Gamma benzene hexachloride (lindane) can cause neurotoxicity through percutaneous absorption, especially in small infants and those with abnormal skin (impetigo, etc), and is, therefore, not recommended in children as first-line therapy for scabies. An excellent alternative—5% permethrin cream (Elimite)—is safer and is more often recommended.

I-33. The answer is c. (*Fauci, pp 1635-1643.*) This patient presents with severe COPD and hypoxemia. Chronic CO_2 retention has blunted his hypercarbic drive to breathe; he is dependent on mild hypoxia to stimulate respiration. An inappropriately high oxygen delivery has decreased even that drive, with resulting acute respiratory acidosis and CO_2 narcosis. However, stopping the oxygen will result in severe hypoxemia. Medroxyprogesterone has only a mild stimulatory effect on the respiratory centers, and is not appropriate therapy in this case. The patient has declared a deteriorating course. Continuing to monitor his status before beginning intervention would probably be fatal. Of the choices listed, the initiation of mechanical ventilation is the only acceptable choice. If the patient's mental status were better, noninvasive ventilation (BiPAP) might be considered. This patient has respiratory (not metabolic) acidosis. Bicarbonate plays no role in this acidosis. The correct therapy is to improve the patient's ventilation.

I-34. The answer is c. (*Katz, pp 148-152. ACOG Guidelines for Women's Health Care, pp 145-158.*) In postmenopausal women, routine screening for colon cancer is recommended with a colonoscopy to be performed every 10 years. Alternatively, flexible sigmoidoscopy can be performed every 5 years along with a yearly fecal occult blood test. Mammography should be performed annually in all women more than 50 years old. Postmenopausal women, who are not on hormone replacement therapy, and all women 65 years or older should be screened for osteoporosis with a DEXA scan to determine bone mineral density. All women who have been sexually active should undergo yearly Pap test screening. After a woman has had three or more consecutive normal Pap smears, the Pap test may be performed less frequently in a low-risk woman. Tuberculosis skin testing need be performed only in individuals with HIV infection, those who have close contact with individuals suspected of having TB, those who are IV drug users, those who are residents of nursing homes or long-term-care facilities, or those who work in a profession that is health care related. This patient does not have any risk factors that would necessitate TB testing.

I-35. The answer is d. (*Fleischer and Ludwig, pp 1761-1799.*) This is a case where **nonaccidental trauma (NAT)** should be considered. A **spiral fracture** of the femur in a non-ambulating child is highly suspicious of NAT. **Metaphyseal corner fractures, fractures of the posterior ribs, sternum scapula or spinous processes, or multiple fractures in various stages of healing may be the only presentation of child abuse.** Any type of trauma that does not fit the mechanism should raise the suspicion and alert the physician. In this case, it is unlikely that the patient was able to fit her leg through the crib rails and break her femur. Although in ambulating children it is not uncommon to have spiral fractures of the femur while running. All states have mandatory reporting of child abuse. According to the AAP (American Academy of Pediatrics), the **skeletal survey** is the initial test of choice for all children suspected of being abused. It is also mandatory to contact the local **Child Protective Services** to further investigate the situation.

Osteogenesis imperfecta (**a**) is a rare genetic condition caused by mutations of the type I procollagen gene. Children may present with fractures in the setting of little or no trauma. Classic blue sclerae may be present. This type of injury (**e**) should not be simply splinted and discharged home. Treatment may consist of a spica cast and close monitoring by orthopedics. For that reason orthopedic surgery (**b**) should be included early in the intervention. Electrolyte abnormalities (**c**) which may be responsible for pathologic fractures in children are exceedingly rare when compared to child abuse and should only be considered once NAT is excluded or in the presence of other abnormalities in the physical examination.

I-36. The answer is e. (*South-Paul, pp 182-189.*) Many medications can cause sexual dysfunction. Medications that commonly cause ejaculatory dysfunction in men include β-blockers, α-blockers, antipsychotics, and

SSRIs. Hydrochlorothiazide can cause erectile dysfunction and decreased libido. Omeprazole and bupropion often do not negatively impact sexual functioning.

1-37. The answer is c. (*Brunicardi, pp 49, 55.*) Magnesium deficiency is common in malnourished patients and patients with large gastrointestinal fluid losses. The neuromuscular effects resemble those of calcium deficiency—namely, paresthesia, hyperreflexia, muscle spasm, and, ultimately, tetany. The cardiac effects are more like those of hypercalcemia. An electrocardiogram therefore provides a rapid means of differentiating between hypocalcemia (prolonged QT interval, T-wave inversion, heart blocks) and hypomagnesemia (prolonged QT and PR intervals, ST segment depression, flattening or inversion of p waves, torsade de pointes). Hypomagnesemia also causes potassium wasting by the kidney. Many hospital patients with refractory hypocalcemia will be found to be magnesium deficient. Often this deficiency becomes manifest during the response to parenteral nutrition when normal cellular ionic gradients are restored. A normal blood pH and arterial $P\text{CO}_2$ rule out hyperventilation. The serum calcium in this patient is normal when adjusted for the low albumin (add 0.8 mg/dL per 1 g/dL decrease in albumin). Hypomagnesemia causes functional hypoparathyroidism, which can lower serum calcium and thus result in a combined defect.

1-38. The answer is d. (*Ropper, pp 783-784.*) This young woman almost certainly has MS. Her visual loss can be explained by optic neuritis, and her bladder problems may be due to demyelination of corticospinal tract fibers. Many patients are reluctant to discuss minor problems with bladder, bowel, or sexual function with a physician of the opposite sex. The positive Babinski sign, focal dysmetria, and apparent dysarthria all support the diagnosis of a multifocal CNS lesion. Multiple lesions disseminated in time and space are typical of MS. With MRI, the multifocal areas of demyelination should be apparent. Many more lesions may be evident on MRI than are suggested by the physical examination.

1-39. The answer is b. (*Aminoff, pp 794-797.*) The clinical scenario presented is most consistent with a neuropathy of Lyme disease, the infection caused by *Borrelia burgdorferi*. This spirochetal infection is tick-borne and is endemic in the area where this patient lives. The rash on his leg was most likely erythema chronicum migrans, a target-shaped lesion that enlarges as the central area returns to normal. His complaints and examination suggest a chronic meningitis preceded by an arthralgia, a common neurologic scenario with Lyme disease. Facial weakness may be the only neurologic sign of Lyme disease. The neurologic deficits usually appear weeks after the initial rash. Untreated neurologic disease may persist for months. Optic neuritis may also appear in association with the chronic meningitis of Lyme disease. A schwannoma may develop on the seventh cranial nerve, but it would produce unilateral facial weakness followed by signs of brainstem compression. The cranial nerve dysfunctions associated with the early stages of diphtheritic polyneuropathy are a consequence of a toxin released by the infectious agent. Tuberculous meningitis may produce several different cranial nerve deficits. With HIV infection, a peripheral neuropathy may develop, but it typically affects the limb nerves, not the facial nerve.

1-40 to 1-46. The answers are 40-d, 41-b, 42-c, 43-a, 44-e, 45-g, 46-f. *(Kaplan, pp 507-508, 510, 1076.)* Persecutory and jealous delusions are probably the most frequently seen by psychiatrists. Patients with the persecutory subtype of delusion are convinced they are being harassed or harmed by others. Those with the jealous type are often verbally and physically abusive to those involved in the delusion (the wife in this case). These delusions are very difficult to treat. The erotomanic delusion consists of the patient believing that someone (usually someone of perceived higher status, like a TV star) is in love with them. Somatic type delusions cause the sufferer to believe that they are afflicted with some physical disorder, and this belief is fixed (unlike hypochondriasis, in which the sufferer can be relieved of the belief that something is wrong, if only temporarily). Grandiose delusions have the patient believing that there is something special about him/her, such as God giving special messages. Mixed delusions combine several types of delusions in one presentation. Unspecified delusions are those reserved for presentations which cannot be characterized by the previous types. One example is Capgras syndrome, which is a delusion in which the patient believes that familiar people have been replaced by imposters.

Block 2

Answers

2-1. The answer is e. (*Rosen, p 1155.*) The **classic triad of aortic stenosis is dyspnea, chest pain, and exertional syncope.** Syncope is a result of either inadequate cerebral perfusion or occasional dysrhythmias. The classic auscultory finding is a **harsh systolic ejection murmur** that is best heard in the second right intercostal space with radiation to the carotid arteries. Syncope in the setting of a new systolic murmur always should raise the suspicion for aortic stenosis as the etiology. The ECG usually reveals **left ventricular hypertrophy.**

(a) Asystole denotes the lack of electrical activity of the heart. Individuals usually don't recover from an asystolic cardiac arrest. (b) Brugada syndrome is caused by an autosomal dominant trait resulting in total loss of function of the cardiac sodium channel or in acceleration of recovery from sodium channel activation. It leads to syncope and may cause sudden cardiac death secondary to a polymorphic ventricular tachycardia. It is associated with a distinctive ECG pattern of downsloping ST-segment elevation in leads V_1 to V_3 with a right bundle-branch block pattern. (c) The subclavian steal syndrome is a rare but important cause of syncope. The syndrome results from occlusion of the proximal subclavian artery and the development of retrograde flow to the subclavian artery from the vertebral artery. (d) A PE that causes syncope usually causes the individual to have unstable vital signs secondary to obstruction of a major vessel.

2-2. The answer is c. (*ACOG, Committee Opinion 321.*) Determination of ethical conduct in doctor—patient relationships can sometimes be very difficult for the physician who is confronted with a patient's autonomy in making a decision that the physician finds incomprehensible. However, the autonomy of the patient who is oriented and alert must be respected even if it means in effect that the patient is committing suicide. The obtaining of a court order to transfuse an adult against his or her will is almost never an acceptable option and leads to a tremendously slippery slope of the doctor's control of the patient's behavior. A patient's spouse also does not have legal authority to make decisions for the patient if the patient is competent, awake, and alert.

The situation is different when a child is involved, and then societal interests can occasionally override parental autonomy. It would be inappropriate for a physician to abandon a patient without obtaining suitable coverage from another qualified physician. Transfusing forcibly is assault and battery; thus, in this case, the physician must adhere to the patient's wishes and, if need be, let her die.

2-3. The answer is d. *(Hay, p 47. Kliegman, pp 1559-1560. McMillan, p 373. Rudolph, pp 1403-1404.)* The finding of polyhydramnios suggests high intestinal obstruction, signs of which include abdominal distention and early and repeated regurgitation. Distention usually is not present, as vomiting keeps the intestine decompressed. The bile-stained vomitus of the infant places the obstruction distal to the ampulla of Vater, eliminating esophageal atresia and pyloric stenosis from consideration. The "double bubble" sign on the x-ray is characteristic of duodenal atresia, which is compatible with the history. Midgut volvulus, which may obstruct the bowel in the area of the duodenojejunal junction, most often produces signs after an affected infant is 3 or 4 days old with acute onset of bilious vomitus. Gastric duplication does not usually produce intestinal obstruction; a cystic mass may be palpated on abdominal examination. Patients with duodenal atresia should be examined closely for evidence of other conditions such as Down syndrome or heart disease.

2-4. The answer is e. *(Fauci, pp 1755, 2492.)* The patient likely has diverticulitis. He is also, however, at high risk of development of radiography-contrast-induced nephropathy from the CT scan. Volume depletion, diabetes mellitus, congestive heart failure, chronic kidney disease and multiple myeloma are all risk factors for contrast-induced kidney damage. The patient's renal risk can be reduced by correction of his volume status with IV fluids. In at-risk patients who are euvolemic, aggressive hydration with normal saline or iso-osmolar sodium bicarbonate infusion prior to and after contrast administration reduces renal damage. Risk may also be decreased by the use of low-osmolar, nonionic contrast agents. N-acetylcysteine is commonly used to decrease the risk of renal damage, but appropriate fluid resuscitation remains paramount. Prophylaxis of venous thromboembolism (VTE) would be important if the patient is hospitalized but would not take precedence over fluid resuscitation. Ischemic colitis is usually caused by low flow in a mesenteric vessel; even if this were the diagnosis (and diverticulitis is more likely), therapeutic doses of anticoagulants are not used in the treatment of ischemic colitis. Aspirin is not acceptable prophylaxis of VTE.

2-5. The answer is a. (*Fauci, pp 1448-1453.*) ACE inhibitors and beta-blockers are the basic regimen for patients with CHF and a depressed ejection fraction. The addition of spironolactone has been shown to be beneficial in management of CHF in patients with New York Heart Association Class III or IV heart failure and an ejection fraction less than 35%. NYHA Class III patients have marked limitation, with symptoms on less than usual activities. NYHA Class IV patients are dyspneic at rest. Although aspirin, warfarin, or amlodipine may be given for other indications, they are unlikely to improve his CHF symptoms. The combination of hydralazine and isosorbide dinitrate has been shown to be advantageous in African Americans who remain symptomatic on ACEIs and beta-blockers.

2-6. The answer is a. (*Kliegman, p 2380. McMillan, p 2650. Rudolph, p 2089.*) The constellation of signs described suggest Noonan syndrome. Other features of this syndrome include cubitus valgus, pulmonary stenosis, edema of the dorsum of the hands and feet, hearing loss, pectus excavatum, bleeding diathesis, and mental retardation in about one-fourth of cases. These patients have many features in common with Turner syndrome, and the condition is often referred to as the "male Turner syndrome," although it occurs in both genders. Inheritance is occasionally autosomal dominant, but is more commonly sporadic.

None of the other choices result in a constellation of signs as described. Mental retardation is a prominent feature of untreated congenital hypothyroidism and Down syndrome, and also would be likely in congenital rubella.

2-7. The answer is d. (*Kaplan, p 206.*) Projection is recognized when a person perceives and reacts to an unacceptable inner impulse as if the impulse were coming from the external environment. In this case, the patient, likely with a huge amount of internal anger that she finds dangerous and unacceptable, projects this anger onto the therapist and reacts as if the therapist is angry at her. Distortion is the reshaping of external reality to suit one's inner needs. For example, a singer who is told at an audition that she needs a lot of work to make her voice stronger remembers the audition as notable for receiving only positive feedback. Blocking is the inhibition of thinking, temporarily and transiently. Isolation is the splitting or separating of an idea from the emotion that accompanies it (but has been repressed). Dissociation is the temporary but drastic modification of a person's sense of personal identity so that emotional distress can be avoided. Fugue states are one example of dissociation in action.

2-8. The answer is b. *(Fauci, p. 2357-2361.)* This young man presents with two obvious serum abnormalities—hypercalcemia and hyperprolactinemia most likely secondary to the pituitary tumor. This, along with his positive family history of a younger sibling with high calcium and low blood sugar and a father who died from an unknown tumor, indicates this family has one of the multiple endocrine neoplasia syndromes. MEN I is associated with parathyroid hyperplasia/adenoma, islet cell hyperplasia/ adenoma/carcinoma, pituitary hyperplasia/adenoma, pheochromocytoma, carcinoid and subcutaneous lipomas. Although MEN 2A is associated with parathyroid hyperplasia/ adenoma, there is no pituitary abnormality with the MEN 2 syndromes (either MEN 2A or MEN 2B). It would not be prudent to treat the patient's issues as two separate abnormalities (primary hyperparathyroidism and prolactinoma). Tension headache is unlikely in the face of a pituitary tumor and visual field deficit.

2-9. The answer is e. *(Brennan, pp 243-246.)* Patient confidentiality demands that you maintain safeguards related to the disclosure of patient information. This is dictated by the patient, even if the wife is the other person in the communication triad.

2-10. The answer is d. *(Townsend, p 2110.)* The CT findings are consistent with any of the suggested lesions. However, the most likely diagnosis in an immunocompetent patient is metastatic disease, which has an incidence of approximately 150,000 to 250,000 cases per year as compared to primary intracranial tumors, which have an incidence of 35,000 per year. Roughly 15% to 30% of cancer patients develop intracranial metastases during the course of their disease. The cancers that most frequently metastasize to the brain parenchyma include those of the lung, breast, kidney, gastrointestinal (GI) tract, and melanomas. Leukemia shows a predilection for the leptomeninges. A large majority of these lesions become symptomatic owing to mass effect from white matter edema. Treatment is dependent on the number and size of the lesions and the physical condition of the patient, but may include a combination of surgery, radiosurgery, and whole-brain radiation therapy. Immunocompromised patients are at increased risk for toxoplasmosis and central nervous system lymphomas. Both immunocompetent and immunocompromised hosts can develop pyogenic brain abscesses, which typically occur in the setting of known infection (which can spread either locally or hematogenously).

2-11. The answer is e. *(South-Paul, pp 310-328.)* Dyspepsia refers to a set of symptoms that can encompass a variety of diseases and the etiologies associated with them. Most clinicians describe dyspepsia as chronic or recurrent discomfort centered around the upper abdomen. Dyspepsia can be associated with heartburn, belching, bloating, nausea, or vomiting, and while common causes include peptic ulcer disease (PUD) and GERD, no specific etiology is found for 50% to 60% of patients who present with dyspepsia. Only 15% to 25% of patients with dyspepsia have ulcer disease, and only 5% to 15% have GERD. Rare causes include gastric or pancreatic cancers.

2-12. The answer is a. *(Ropper, pp 16-18.)* Computed tomographic scanning measures the density of intracranial as well as extracranial structures. Bone appears much denser than blood, but blood is obvious on the unenhanced (precontrast) CT scan precisely because it is much denser than white matter, gray matter, and CSF. The resolution of the CT scan is generally not sufficient to differentiate the pia mater from the gray matter on which it lies. Other meningeal structures, such as the dura mater, may appear denser than brain, especially if there is some calcification in the membranes.

2-13. The answer is d. *(Kaplan, p 476.)* Factors weighting toward a good prognosis in schizophrenia include: late onset of the disease, obvious precipitating factors/stressors, an acute onset, good premorbid functioning, the presence of mood disorder symptoms, the patient being married, a family history of mood disorders, good support systems, and the presence of positive symptoms (as opposed to negative symptoms).

2-14. The answer is a. *(Tintinalli, pp 328-331.)* Direct sun exposure during healing can lead to permanent hyperpigmentation. Therefore, **avoiding direct sun exposure** and using sun block for up to 12 months can improve cosmetic outcome.
(**b**) Patients should be instructed to wash the wound with gentle soap and water as early as 8 hours after sutures are placed. Although the wound should be kept dry, instructing against washing is inappropriate. Healing wounds should be patted dry to avoid dehiscence from forceful wiping. (**e**) The patient should be informed that all lacerations scar. Good repair and wound care will improve the appearance of the scar but will not inhibit scar formation. Wounds that heal by delayed closure have the poorest cosmetic outcome. Good edge approximation, using appropriate suture material, and early suture removal all lead to better cosmetic outcomes. (**d**) The early appearance of the scar is not reflective of the long-term outcome. (**c**) Facial sutures should be removed in 3 to 5 days. Leaving sutures in for 7 to 10 days lead to a poorer outcome.

2-15. The answer is e. *(Ropper, pp 158-159.)* The headache is typical of that caused by intracranial hypertension. Additionally, the patient has focal neurological symptoms and signs. This creates particular concern about a brain tumor or hemorrhage, and the patient should be evaluated as soon as possible. An appointment next month is too late. Intravenous prochlorperazine is a good treatment for status migrainosus; however, this history is atypical for such a diagnosis, and more serious problems should be ruled out first in the emergency room. Zolmitriptan is a treatment for migraines. This history is not typical for migraine, and zolmitriptan is also relatively contraindicated in patients with complex migraine. This history is very atypical for seizures, and an electroencephalogram is not likely to provide useful information in this case.

2-16. The answer is c. *(Hay, pp 860-862. Kliegman, pp 2082-2084. McMillan, pp 1731-1733. Rudolph, pp 1556-1557.)* In children, ITP is the most common form of thrombocytopenic purpura. In most cases, a preceding viral infection can be noted. No diagnostic test identifies this disease; exclusion of the other diseases listed in the question is necessary. In this disease, the platelet count is frequently less than 20,000/μL, but other laboratory tests yield essentially normal results, including the bone marrow aspiration (if done). Complications are uncommon; significant bleeding occurs in only 5% of cases and intracranial hemorrhage is even rarer. The treatment of childhood ITP is controversial. Patients with mild symptoms such as bruising and self-limited epistaxis may be observed, while patients with significant bleeding should be treated. IVIG and corticosteroids are effective in causing a rapid increase in platelet count, but controversy exists surrounding the use of prednisone before ruling out leukemia with a bone marrow aspirate. For Rh-positive patients with a working spleen, the use of anti-D immunoglobulin also results in an increase in platelet count. For patients with chronic (> 1 year) ITP, a splenectomy may be helpful.

Aplastic anemia is unlikely if the other cell lines are normal. Von Willebrand disease might be expected to present with bleeding and not just bruising. It is unlikely that acute leukemia would present with thrombocytopenia only. Thrombotic thrombocytopenic purpura is rare in children.

2-17. The answer is c. *(McPhee, pp 637-639.)* The history and physical described are classic for trichomonas vaginalis. The classic "strawberry cervix" is a strong diagnostic clue. Trichomonads are seen on high power in the saline preparation, and appear as triangular cells with long tails, slightly larger than WBC. "Studded" epithelial cells (clue cells) are more consistent with bacterial vaginosis, "moth-eaten" cells (pseudo-clue cells) are seen in an acid-base disturbance of the vagina. Numerous WBC are more consistent with an upper genital infection, and hyphae are consistent with vaginal candidiasis.

2-18. The answer is e. *(Ropper, pp 910-913.)* Writhing and jerking movements of the limbs are part of the chorea that typically develops with Huntington disease. Dopaminergic drugs, such as L-dopa, bromocriptine, and lisuride, may unmask chorea. This is inadvisable as a diagnostic technique because it may contribute to the premature symptom of chorea. Dopamine antagonists, such as haloperidol, may be used to suppress chorea, but also carry the risk of provoking tardive dyskinesia. Huntington disease is characterized pathologically by loss of several neuronal types in the striatum (caudate and putamen). It has been hypothesized that the occurrence of dopaminergic-induced chorea in Huntington disease is related to increased sensitivity of the dopamine receptors in the remaining striatal neurons, although there are abnormalities in several other neurotransmitters as well. Choreiform movements develop in a variety of other conditions; the one most similar to Huntington disease is hereditary acanthocytosis.

2-19. The answer is c. *(Greenfield, pp 183-187.)* By far the most likely cause of the oliguria observed in this patient is hypovolemia. Volume status would be best assessed by placing a Swan-Ganz catheter to measure the preload pressures in the left atrium (by inference from the pulmonary capillary wedge pressures). Patients who undergo long, difficult operations in large surgical fields collect third-space fluids and become intravascularly depleted despite large volumes of intravenous fluid and blood replacement. The proper management usually involves titrating the cardiac output by providing as much fluid as necessary to keep the wedge pressures near 15 mm Hg. The other studies listed might become useful if urinary flow remains depressed after optimal cardiac output has been achieved, but in view of the probability of hypovolemia, they are not indicated as first diagnostic studies.

2-20. The answer is c. *(Tintinalli, pp 1547-1551.)* **Crohn disease** is characterized by **chronic inflammation extending through all layers of the bowel wall.** Onset is generally between the ages of 15 and 40 years. Crohn disease should be suspected in any patient whose symptoms show a picture consistent with chronic inflammatory colitis. Extraintestinal manifestations are seen in 25% to 30% of patients. The incidence is similar for Crohn disease and ulcerative colitis. They include aphthous ulcers, erythema nodosum, iritis or episcleritis, arthritis, and gallstones. **Nephrolithiasis** is seen as a result of hyperoxaluria because of increased oxalate absorption in patients with ileal disease. Because ulcerative colitis affects only the large bowel, this extraintestinal manifestation is seen only in patients with Crohn disease.

2-21. The answer is d. (*Fauci, pp 1695-1702.*) This patient is septic, and immediate therapy should be directed at correcting her hemodynamic instability. Patients with sepsis require aggressive fluid resuscitation to compensate for capillary extravasation. This patient's vital signs suggest decreased effective circulating volume. Normal saline at 100 cc/h is insufficient volume replacement. The patient should be given a saline bolus of 2 L over 20 minutes, and then her blood pressure and clinical status should be reassessed. The elevated respiratory rate could be evidence of pulmonary edema or respiratory compensation of acidosis from decreased tissue perfusion. Even if the patient has evidence of pulmonary edema, fluid resuscitation remains the first intervention for hypotension from sepsis. She is more likely to die from hemodynamic collapse than from oxygenation issues related to pulmonary edema.

Stress doses of hydrocortisone and intravenous norepinephrine are both used in patients with shock refractory to volume resuscitation, but should be reserved until after the saline bolus. Vancomycin is a reasonable choice to cover enterococci, which can cause UTI-associated sepsis, but again would not address the immediate hemodynamic problem. If the patient does not improve, a central line (to measure filling pressures and mixed venous oxygen saturation) would allow the "early goal-directed" sepsis protocol to be used.

2-22. The answer is e. (*Kaplan, pp 949-953.*) Biofeedback refers to a therapeutic process in which information about the individual's physiological functions, such as blood pressure and heart rate, are monitored electronically and fed back to the individual by means of lights, sounds, or electronic gauges. Biofeedback allows individuals to control a variety of body responses and in turn to modulate pain and the physiological component of unpleasant emotions such as anxiety.

2-23. The answer is c. (*Katz, pp 576-578, 744-748.*) The human papillomaviruses (HPV) are a group of double-stranded DNA viruses that infect epithelial cells. They do not cause systemic infection. There are numerous viruses within the group, and they are named by number according to the order of their discovery. Human papilloma viruses are sexually transmitted. HPV, in particular types 16, 18, and 31, have been linked to cervical neoplasia. HPV types 6 and 11 are associated with benign condyloma.

2-24. The answer is a. *(Tintinalli, p 1077.)* Patients with chest pain in the setting of cocaine use should be evaluated for possible myocardial ischemia. Patients suspected of ACS should be managed accordingly with oxygen, nitrates, morphine, aspirin, and benzodiazepines; however, **β-adrenergic antagonist** therapy is **absolutely contraindicated.** If β-adrenergic receptors are antagonized, α-adrenergic receptors are left unopposed and available for increased stimulation by cocaine. This may worsen into coronary and peripheral vasoconstriction, hypertension, and possibly ischemia. Therefore, benzodiazepines, which decrease central sympathetic outflow, are the cornerstone in treatment to relieve cocaine-related chest pain.

(**b**) Diltiazem, a CCB, can be used in patients with cocaine-related chest pain. It is used to lower HR. (**c**) Aspirin should be administered to all patients with chest pain, unless there is a contraindication. In patients with cocaine-related chest pain who also seize, aspirin may be held until a CT scan is performed to rule out an intracranial bleed. (**d**) Lorazepam, a benzodiazepine, is an excellent medication to use in cocaine-related chest pain as it reduces their sympathetic drive leading to a reduction in BP and HR. (**e**) Nitroglycerin should be administered to these patients if they have chest pain. Nitrates dilate the coronary arteries, increasing blood flow to the myocardium.

2-25. The answer is d. *(American Academy of Family Physicians, 2008.)* There is a strong recommendation from the American Academy of Family Physicians for cervical cancer screening at least every 3 years for women who have ever had sex and have a cervix. However, the optimal age at which to begin screening is unknown. Some recommend that screening should start at the onset of sexual activity or at age 18, whichever comes first. However, evidence, coupled with the natural history of HPV infection, indicates that screening can safely be delayed until 3 years after the onset of sexual activity or age 21, whichever comes first.

2-26. The answer is d. *(Hay, pp 22-23. Kliegman, pp 720-721. Rudolph, p 89.)* Infants born to mothers with gestational diabetes are at risk for being large for their gestational age and thus at increased risk for peripheral nerve injuries such as Erb-Duchenne and phrenic nerve paralysis. An ultrasound or fluoroscopy of the chest would reveal asymmetric diaphragmatic motion in a seesaw manner. With a negative chest radiograph, a chest CT would not be helpful at this point. Bronchoscopy would help delineate airway abnormalities and foreign bodies, but would not identify phrenic nerve paralysis.

2-27. The answer is d. *(Patten, pp 256-257.)* A syrinx is an abnormal fluid collection resulting in an expansion of the central canal. As the lesion in this region of the spinal cord increases in size, it may affect the lower motor neuron in the anterior horn of the spinal cord, producing weakness in the distribution of the affected motor neurons. Because it is a lower motor neuron lesion, reflexes will be lost rather than increased in the upper extremities, which may at first seem counterintuitive in a spinal cord lesion. The more laterally placed corticospinal tract may be spared, leaving leg function and reflexes relatively normal. Charcot joints are the result of cumulative damage from loss of reflexes and diminished pain awareness, classically associated with syphilis or more commonly diabetes.

2-28. The answer is c. *(Greenfield, pp 139-140.)* TNF is a peptide hormone produced by endotoxin-activated monocytes/macrophages and has been postulated to be the principal cytokine mediator in gram-negative shock and sepsis-related organ damage. Biologic actions of TNF include polymorphonuclear neutrophil (PMN) activation and degranulation; increased nonspecific host resistance; increased vascular permeability; lymphopenia; promotion of interleukins 1, 2, and 6; capillary leak syndrome; microvascular thrombosis; anorexia and cachexia; and numerous other protective and adverse effects in sepsis. Its role in sepsis provides a fertile field for research in critical care.

2-29. The answer is e. *(Hay, pp 90-92. Kliegman, pp 2476-2477. Rudolph, p 2274.)* The child in this question most likely has breath-holding spells. Two forms exist. Cyanotic spells consist of the symptoms outlined and are predictable upon upsetting or scolding the child. They are rare before 6 months of age, peak at about 2 years of age, and resolve by about 5 years of age. Avoidance of reinforcing this behavior is the treatment of choice. Pallid breath-holding spells are less common and are usually caused by a painful experience (such as a fall). With these events, the child will stop breathing, lose consciousness, become pale and hypotonic, and may have a brief tonic episode. Although the family may be concerned that these "tonic episodes" are seizures, the temporal relationship with an inciting event make this diagnosis highly unlikely. These pallid events, too, resolve spontaneously. Again, avoidance of reinforcing behavior is indicated. Assuring the family that this is a benign condition is important.

2-30. The answer is b. *(Ropper, p 788.)* Clinical trials have shown that intravenous methylprednisolone for an attack of optic neuritis is associated

with a better outcome than oral prednisone. Intravenous methylprednisolone is thus recommended by most experts as appropriate therapy for
acute exacerbations of MS involving more than sensory manifestations alone.

2-31. The answer is b. (*Moore and Jefferson, pp 191-205.*) In adolescents
and young adults, gender identity disorder is characterized by strong cross-
gender identification, a persistent discomfort with one's sex, and clinically
significant distress or impairment. Such patients usually trace their convic-
tion to early childhood, often live as the opposite sex, and seek sex reassignment surgery and endocrine treatment. These patients feel a sense of relief
and appropriateness when they are wearing opposite-sex clothing. In contrast, patients with transvestic fetishism are sexually aroused by this behavior, and so typically only seek to wear clothing of the opposite sex during
sexual situations. Homosexuality is not a diagnosis in DSM-IV. While some
homosexuals cross-dress to seek a same-sex partner, they do not feel that
they belong to the opposite sex, nor do they seek sex reassignment surgery.

2-32. The answer is d. (*Ransom, pp 172-174.*) Puerperal mastitis may be
subacute, but is often characterized by chills, fever, and tachycardia. If undiagnosed, it may progress to suppurative mastitis with abscess formation that
requires drainage. The most common offending organism is *Staphylococcus
aureus,* which is probably transmitted from the infant's nose and throat. A
culture of the breast milk should be done prior to initiation of antibiotic therapy. Dicloxacillin, a penicillinase-resistant antibiotic, is the initial treatment
of choice. In penicillin-allergic patients, erythromycin is recommended.
Treatment should last for 7 to 10 days. If a mass is palpable, an abscess
should be suspected. Incision and drainage is recommended for a breast
abscess. The patient should continue to breast-feed on the affected breast; if
it is too painful she may pump. After antibiotic therapy is initiated, the
patient should be reevaluated to ensure improvement.

2-33. The answer is c. (*Mengel, pp 593-603.*) Most clinicians agree that
psychiatric disorders cannot be reliably assessed in patients who are currently or recently intoxicated. Alcohol is a depressant, and may be the main
factor in the patient's depressive symptoms. Detoxification and a period of
abstinence are necessary before an evaluation for other psychiatric disorders can be effectively completed.

2-34. The answer is d. (*McQuaid, pp 285-316.*) Omeprazole (Prilosec)
irreversibly inhibits the hydrogen-potassium-ATPase (proton pump) in the

secretory canaliculus of the gastric parietal cell. This blocks the last step in the acid-secretory process. Omeprazole's duration of action exceeds 24 hours, and doses of 20 to 30 mg/day inhibit more than 90% of 24-hour acid secretion. Omeprazole provides excellent suppression of meal-stimulated and nocturnal acid secretion and seems very safe for short-term therapy. Prolonged administration in laboratory animals has been associated with significant hypergastrinemia, hyperplasia of enterochromaffin-like cells, and carcinoid tumors.

2-35. The answer is d. (*Kaplan, p 477.*) Catatonic schizophrenia is characterized by marked psychomotor disturbances including prolonged immobility, posturing, extreme negativism (the patient actively resists any attempts made to change his or her position) or waxy flexibility (the patient maintains the position in which he or she is placed), mutism, echolalia (repetition of words said by another person), and echopraxia (repetition of movements made by another person). Periods of immobility and mutism can alternate with periods of extreme agitation (catatonic excitement).

2-36. The answer is c. (*Mengel, pp 132-136.*) There are many medications known to cause peripheral edema as a side effect. Antihypertensives, such as calcium channel blockers are well-known to cause this, but direct vasodilators, β-blockers, centrally acting agents, and antisympathetics also can cause edema. Of the diabetic medications, insulin sensitizers, such as rosiglitazone often cause edema. Hormones, corticosteroids, and NSAIDs also cause problems. SSRIs like fluoxetine do not commonly cause this symptom. Neither do ACE inhibitors, like lisinopril, or thiazide diuretics.

2-37. The answer is b. (*Tintinalli, pp 1389-1390.*) The CT depicts subarachnoid arachnoid blood. This patient may have had a sentinel bleed, a small SAH, the previous week. Noncontrast CT misses a small percentage of SAH and therefore, in cases of high suspicion, an LP must be obtained to exclude the diagnosis.

Irritation of the meninges or inflammation of the brain (**a**) may not appear at all on noncontrast CT of the brain. If contrast is used, meningeal or cerebral enhancement may be apparent, but diagnosis of these conditions is not based on imaging. High clinical suspicion must be present for either condition and LP is used to confirm the diagnosis. Hydrocephalus (**c**) appears as dilated ventricles on CT scan. If all of the ventricles are patent and dilated, it is termed communicating hydrocephalus. If part of the ventricular system is collapsed and the others dilated, an obstructive cause of hydrocephalus is present. Epidural hematomas (**d**) are the result of brisk arterial bleeds into the space between the dura and the calvarium. They are classically caused by trauma and are associated with a "lucid period" during which level of consciousness is normal prior to neurologic deterioration. On noncontrast CT, they appear as hyperdense intracranial collections of blood that are bilenticular in shape. Subdural hematomas (SDH) (**e**) are intracranial blood collections that result from tearing of the bridging veins between the dura and the brain. Risk factors for SDH include advanced age and chronic alcohol use. Both conditions are associated with decreased brain volume and provide stretch on these delicate veins. On noncontrast CT, SDHs appear as crescent shaped collections of hyperdense blood.

2-38.   The answer is e. (*Kliegman, pp 2443-2444. McMillan, p 266. Rudolph, p 2185.*) The child in the photograph has a hairy nevus over the spine; virtually any abnormality (except Mongolian spots) over the lower spine points to the possibility of occult spinal dysraphism. This designation includes a number of spinal cord and vertebral anomalies that frequently produce severe loss of neurologic function, particularly in the region of the back, the lower extremities, and the urinary system. Examples of these abnormalities are subcutaneous lipomeningomyelocele, diastematomyelia, hamartoma, lipoma, tight filum terminale, tethered cord, dermal and epidermal cysts, dermal sinuses, neurenteric canals, and angiomas. Occasionally, the loss of neurologic function from such anomalies is mild and, as a result, easily overlooked. Prompt evaluation of these lesions via CT, MRI, or ultrasound is indicated. Epstein pearls are benign, small, white lesions noted on a newborn's hard palate. Mongolian spots are flat, hyperpigmented lesions on the lower back, buttocks, and occasionally elsewhere; they are more common on blacks, Hispanic, and Asian children and are not pathologic (although they are sometimes confused for bruising by the inexperienced observer). A cephalohematoma is a subperiosteal collection of blood that does not cross the suture line found on a newborn's scalp. Omphalocele, extravasations of intestinal contents into an abdominal wall sac, would be noted on the ventral surface.

2-39 to 2-41.   The answers are 39-f, 40-d, 41-b. (*Fauci, pp 2053-2061.*) C1 inhibitor deficiency prevents the proper regulation of activated C1. As a consequence, levels of C2 and C4—-substrates of C1—-are also low. Recurrent angioedema is the result of uncontrolled action of other serum proteins normally controlled by C1 inhibitor. The disease may be acquired but is usually inherited in an autosomal dominant pattern as a result of a deficiency of C1 inhibitor. There is no pruritus or urticarial lesions. Recurrent gastrointestinal attacks of colic commonly occur.

Immunoglobulin A deficiency is the commonest immunodeficiency syndrome, occurring in 1 in 600 patients. It is especially common in Caucasians. The most well-defined aspect of the syndrome is the development of severe allergic reactions to the IgA contained in transfused blood. Patients probably have an increased incidence of sinopulmonary infections and chronic diarrheal illness, although the increased susceptibility may be attributed to concomitant IgG subclass (especially IgG2 and IgG4) deficiency. There is no effective treatment for the IgA deficiency although those with IgG subclass deficiency and recurrent bacterial infections may benefit from immunoglobulin infusions.

Ataxia-telangiectasia is an uncommon genetic syndrome of immunodeficiency, cerebellar ataxia, and facial and ocular telangiectasias. The patients have abnormal DNA repair and suffer from an increased incidence of cancer, especially lymphomas. The abnormal gene is called the ATM gene; approximately 1% of the population is deficient in one allele. Interestingly, heterozygotes, although otherwise normal, are susceptible to increased radiation damage because of the abnormal DNA repair mechanism.

2-42 to 2-46. The answers are 42-f, 43-c, 44-a, 45-b, 46-e. (*Fauci, pp 2119-2132.*) The large vessel vasculitides include temporal (giant cell) arteritis and Takayasu arteritis. Temporal arteritis typically occurs in older patients and is accompanied by aching in the shoulders and hips, jaw claudication, and a markedly elevated ESR. Takayasu arteritis, a granulomatous inflammation of the aorta and its main branches, typically occurs in young women. Symptoms are attributed to local vascular occlusion and may produce arm or leg claudication. Systemic symptoms of arthralgia, fatigue, malaise, anorexia, and weight loss may precede the vascular symptoms. Surgery may be necessary to correct occlusive lesions.

The patient in question 2-42 has classic polyarteritis nodosa. It is a multisystem necrotizing medium-size vessel vasculitis that, prior to the use of steroids and cyclophosphamide, was uniformly fatal. Patients commonly present with signs of vascular insufficiency in the involved organs. Abdominal involvement is common. In 30% of patients, antecedent hepatitis B virus infection can be demonstrated; immune complexes containing the virus have been found in such patients and are likely pathogenic.

Small vessel vasculitides include Wegener granulomatosis, microscopic polyangitis, the Churg-Strauss syndrome, Henoch-Schönlein purpura, and cryoglobulinemic vasculitis. Wegener granulomatosis usually involves the sinuses, lungs, and kidneys. CXR may reveal cavities, infiltrates, or nodules. Many patients also develop glomerulonephritis which may result in acute renal failure. On biopsy, the vasculitis is necrotizing and granulomatous. Microscopic polyangiitis is a multisystem necrotizing vasculitis that typically results in glomerulonephritis, pulmonary hemorrhage, and fever. Lung biopsy shows inflammation of capillaries. Patients may also have mononeuritis multiplex and palpable purpura. Classic polyarteritis nodosa rarely involves the lungs.

The Churg-Strauss syndrome is characterized by wheezing, fever, eosinophilia and systemic vasculitis that may involve the peripheral nerves, central nervous system, heart, kidneys, or GI tract. Henoch-Schönlein purpura primarily occurs in children and presents with palpable purpura, arthritis, and glomerulonephritis. A third of the affected children will have a glomerulonephritis which occasionally results in renal failure. Cryoglobulinemia can be associated with a small vessel vasculitis. Patients typically present with palpable purpura, arthritis, and glomerulonephritis. Cryoglobulinemia is often associated with hepatitis C.

Block 3

Answers

3-1. The answer is d. *(Rosen, pp 381-383.)* Given the history of trauma, a **rib fracture** is the most probable etiology of the patient's symptoms in this clinical scenario. Rib fractures usually occur at the **point of impact** or at the **posterior angle**, which is the weakest part of the rib. It is important to note that the true danger of rib fractures involves not the rib itself, but the risk of penetrating injury to underlying structures. A **rib series** is the most effective way to visualize these fractures. Treatment of patients with simple acute rib fractures includes pain relief so that respiratory splinting does not occur, which increases the rate of atelectasis and pneumonia. Chest binders should not be used as they promote hypoventilation. For multiple rib fractures, intercostal nerve blocks may be a more effective means of analgesia. Most rib fractures heal uneventfully within 3 to 6 weeks. The patient should be encouraged to take deep breaths to avoid developing pneumonia.

A chest radiograph **(a)** is valuable for investigating other associated injuries, but often obscures the ribs and fractures may remain hidden. A chest CT scan **(b)** is not indicated at this time and is only warranted with worsening symptoms or negative radiographs with a high clinical suspicion. An ECG **(c)** may be obtained to evaluate the general health of this patient but is not helpful in diagnosing a rib fracture. A thoracentesis **(e)**, whether diagnostic or therapeutic, is indicated only in patients with pleural effusions.

3-2. The answer is d. *(Townsend, pp 1923-1924.)* The patient has ischemia of the left colon and rectum. Intestinal ischemia develops when a patent inferior mesenteric artery is ligated in the setting of superior mesenteric artery (SMA) or bilateral hypogastric artery occlusion. Ligation of the IMA too far from the aorta can also interfere with the collateral blood supply to the rectosigmoid and lead to ischemia. Abdominal distention, fever, elevation of white blood cell count, and/or bloody diarrhea in the postoperative period should raise suspicion for colon ischemia. The best study to evaluate the sigmoid and rectum is sigmoidoscopy. Barium enema is not as accurate as sigmoidoscopy in determining depth of injury and carries grave risks of contamination by barium and feces if perforation occurs. CT, MRI, and aortography are not useful in evaluating the colon for early ischemia.

3-3. The answer is a. *(Hay, p 618. Kliegman, pp 1644-1650. McMillan, pp 1925-1927. Rudolph, p 1742.)* A congenital indirect inguinal hernia is the result of a patent processus vaginalis. This is in contrast to the less common acquired direct inguinal hernia, caused by weakness in the musculature of the inguinal canal. Inguinal hernias are commonly seen in premature infants (16%-25%). Incarceration is common; elective repair is often considered prior to hospital discharge. The diagnosis is so common that diagnostic tests are performed infrequently.

3-4. The answer is a. *(Kaplan, pp 467-468, 475.)* Frieda Fromm-Reichmann followed the interpersonal school founded by Harry Stack Sullivan and believed that schizophrenia was the outcome of an inadequate mother–child relationship in which the mother was aloof, overly protective, or hostile. She postulated that faulty mothering leads to anxiety and distrust of others, causing people who develop schizophrenia to withdraw from interpersonal exchanges. This theory has been discredited by recent research that supports the notion that schizophrenia is a brain disorder caused by the convergence of multiple environmental and genetic factors. However, subsequent study of the effect of expressed emotion (family members expressive of hostility and overly controlling) do show that this behavior leads to an increase in relapse rates.

3-5. The answer is b. *(Rakel, pp 918-924.)* Long-acting β-agonists are less effective if not paired with inhaled corticosteroids. A leukotriene receptor antagonist is a better choice in this case. Cromolyn therapy has been replaced by newer agents, mainly because of compliance issues. Theophylline and oral steroids would not be indicated in this case.

3-6. The answer is c. *(Ropper, pp 771-790.)* Patients with a multiple sclerosis often develop a spastic (upper motor neuron) bladder. There is little or no residual urine in the bladder after emptying because bladder contractility is good, but distensibility is poor. The bladder does not distend substantially because of corticospinal tract disease, which produces spasticity. The patient usually has urgency or incontinence.

3-7. The answer is c. *(Townsend, pp 2090-2094.)* The cerebral perfusion pressure is calculated as the difference between the MAP and the ICP;

optimally the CPP should be maintained at greater than 70 mm Hg and the ICP at less than 20 mm Hg. Methods for reducing ICP include elevation of the head of the bed (reverse Trendelenburg), administration of mannitol or other diuretics to improve cerebral blood flow, use of short-acting sedatives to decrease patient agitation (the drugs should be intermittently held to perform neurological examinations), prevention of hypovolemia and treatment of hypotension, and prevention of hypoventilation and hypercapnia. Hypoventilation and hypercapnia cause vasodilation of the cerebral vessels, which increases the intracranial volume and pressure. Hyperventilation may still be used in cases of herniation or impending herniation to acutely lower ICP. However, prolonged hyperventilation is not recommended because of decreased perfusion (secondary to vasoconstriction) to an already ischemic brain. Furthermore, the brain resets to the new target PCO_2 within 48 to 72 hours, limiting the beneficial effects of hyperventilation and resulting in increased ICP when the P_{CO_2} is later normalized. Therefore, hypercarbia should be avoided but hypocapnia below 30 mm Hg cannot be recommended except in extreme circumstances. Use of pressors to maintain a CPP above 70 mm Hg is controversial.

3-8. The answer is d. *(Rosen, pp 1549-1583.)* This patient is experiencing a **visual hallucination,** most typical of a medical rather than psychiatric etiology. **Digoxin** is a common precipitant of these symptoms and may begin with yellow-blue changes in vision, known as van Gogh vision. Digoxin directly binds the Na-K ATPase which increases sodium and calcium levels, increasing the contractility of the heart. Hallucinations are often an early symptom of digoxin overdose. Treatment for this includes a protein fragment that binds this medication.

(a) Auditory hallucinations are usually seen in psychiatric illness or an acute psychotic episode. Antidepressants (e) typically do not produce changes in vision or hallucinations. His symptoms are also not typical of malingering (b), given that he was not brought in of his own accord without secondary gain, or of conversion disorder (c).

3-9. The answer is c. *(Fauci, pp 1632-1635.)* Patients with cystic fibrosis are now surviving into adulthood. The median survival is approximately age 41. Most cases are diagnosed in childhood; however, because of variable penetration of the genetic defect, approximately 7% are not found until the patient is an adult. Most male patients (>95%) are azoospermic. Chronic pulmonary infections occur, and bronchiectasis frequently develops. Diabetes mellitus and gastrointestinal problems indicate pancreatic insufficiency. COPD or emphysema at this age would be unusual unless the patient was deficient in $alpha_1$ antitrypsin. The patient's course is too prolonged for a simple upper respiratory tract infection. He has provided no history of hemoptysis or anemia to suggest a pulmonary hemorrhage syndrome. Asthma would not cause the abdominal symptoms, diabetes, or changes of bronchiectasis.

3-10. The answer is c. (*Moore and Jefferson, pp 138-139.*) The SSRIs, including fluoxetine, paroxetine, sertraline, fluvoxamine, and citalopram are well tolerated by the elderly, as are unique agents such as bupropion, venlafaxine, nefazodone, and mirtazapine. The tricyclic drugs include imipramine, desipramine, amitriptyline, and nortriptyline. They are effective in the treatment of depression; several anxiety disorders including panic disorder, generalized anxiety disorder, and separation anxiety; enuresis; and ADHD. Tricyclic antidepressants have different side effect profiles, with each blocking cholinergic, adrenergic, and histaminic receptors to different degrees. For example, there is less anticholinergic activity with desipramine than with imipramine, and nortriptyline is less likely to cause orthostatic hypotension than amitriptyline. However, all tricyclics are at least somewhat anticholinergic and sedating, and thus should not be used as a first-line treatment for major depression in the elderly. Phenelzine and tranylcypromine are both MAO inhibitors, whose major side effect is hypotension—again, not something to be used in the geriatric population, if at all possible.

3-11. The answer is e. (*South-Paul, pp 13-20.*) Hospital admission is indicated for failure to thrive, in the face of hypotension and bradycardia. These are signs of severe malnutrition. Other interventions may be appropriate, but with vital sign abnormalities, it is important to admit the patient. Patients like this are generally not neglected, especially since he has been seen all along for well-child checks.

3-12. The answer is b. (*Fauci, pp 2513-2531.*) This patient presents with an acute left middle cerebral artery stroke. Time is of the essence if thrombolytic therapy is to be beneficial. Intravenous thrombolytics may be administered up to 3 hours after the onset of symptoms. Fortunately, this patient was brought to the ER promptly. CT scan of the brain shows no evidence of bleed. Evidence of ischemia may not become apparent until 48-72 hours. A prior history of intracranial hemorrhage, recent surgery, bleeding diathesis, onset of symptoms greater than 3 hours prior to therapy and unknown time of onset of symptoms are contraindications to thrombolytic therapy. This patient should be given intravenous tissue-type plasminogen activator (t-PA).

Anticoagulation in acute stroke (answer a) is not currently recommended. In most trials of anticoagulation, any benefit of therapy is matched by an increase in hemorrhagic transformation. Interferon-beta (answer c) is used to treat multiple sclerosis, not ischemic stroke. Emergent scanning with MRI (answer d) wastes precious time and is not always available. Patients with acute stroke often have mild elevation in cardiac biomarkers. Cardiac catheterization (answer e) is unnecessary, and may very well prove harmful in the setting of a stroke.

3-13. The answer is c. (*Hay, pp 868-869. Kliegman, pp 2080-2081. McMillan, pp 1745-1746. Rudolph, p 1575.*) In disseminated intravascular coagulation (DIC), there is consumption of fibrinogen; factors II, V, and VIII; and platelets. Therefore, there is prolongation of PT, aPTT, and TT and a decrease in factor VIII level and platelet count. In addition, the titer of fibrin split production is usually increased. D-dimer is a fibrin breakdown product and may also be elevated in DIC.

The prolongation of PT, aPTT, and TT excludes the diagnosis of ITP. PT tests principally for factors I, II, V, VII, and X and is not prolonged in hemophilia A (factor VIII deficiency) or hemophilia B (factor IX deficiency). In vitamin K deficiency, there is a decrease in the production of factors II, VII, IX, and X, and PT and aPTT are prolonged. The thrombin time, which tests for conversion of fibrinogen to fibrin, however, should be normal, and the platelet count should also be normal.

3-14. The answer is d. (*Roberts and Hedges, pp 562-563.*) The **mental nerve** is a continuation of the inferior alveolar nerve. It emerges from the mental foramen below the second premolar and **innervates the mucosa and skin of the lower lip.** A mental nerve block is the most appropriate way to anesthetize this patient given his lip swelling.

(c) Local injection with lidocaine will cause further swelling and distort the anatomy further. A mental block will provide anesthesia without distorting the lip anatomy. **(e)** The block should be performed with a 25- or 27-gauge needle. An 18-gauge needle is too large for the procedure. The mental foramen should be palpated with a gloved finger. It is located 1-cm inferior and anterior to the second premolar. Lidocaine should be injected around the foramen. **(a)** Injecting directly into the foramen should be avoided because it can cause neurovascular damage. **(b)** This patient will require bilateral mental blocks because his laceration crosses the midline.

3-15. The answer is c. (*Swaiman, pp 784-786.*) The association of erythrocytosis with cerebellar signs, microscopic hematuria, and hepato-splenomegaly suggests von Hippel-Lindau syndrome. This hereditary disorder is characterized by polycystic liver disease, polycystic kidney disease, retinal angiomas (telangiectasia), and cerebellar tumors. This is an autosomal dominant inherited disorder with variable penetrance. Men are more commonly affected than women. Although neoplastic cysts may develop in the cerebellum in persons with von Hippel-Lindau syndrome, these usually do not become sufficiently large to cause an obstructive hydrocephalus. Other abnormalities that occur with this syndrome include adenomas in many organs. Hemangiomas may be evident in the bones, adrenals, and ovaries. Hemangioblastomas may develop in the spinal cord or brainstem, as well as in the cerebellum. This syndrome is not associated with acoustic schwannomas that could cause bilateral hearing loss, and it is not accompanied by peripheral neuropathy, which could cause diffuse hyporeflexia.

3-16. The answer is e. (*Cunningham, pp 763-765, 781-785, 794.*) Hypertension is diagnosed in pregnancy when the resting blood pressure is 140/90 mm Hg or greater. The patient may have a history of chronic hypertension. Gestational hypertension is diagnosed if the patient develops hypertension without proteinuria during the pregnancy. Preeclampsia is diagnosed when the hypertension is associated with proteinuria of greater than 300 mg in a 24 hour collection or persistent 1+ proteinuria in random urine sampling. The cure for gestational hypertension and preeclampsia is delivery. Select preterm patients may be managed conservatively at home or in the hospital depending upon the severity of the hypertension. BPP testing is useful when following the patient conservatively. Although bed rest may transiently improve elevated blood pressure, a patient at full term should be delivered. Based on the severity of this patient's blood pressure and the 4+ proteinuria, she has severe preeclamsia and she should be delivered. Since this patient's fetus is breech, cesarean delivery rather than induction of labor is the next best step in the management of this patient. Diuretics should not be used in the management of preeclampsia, as they deplete the maternal intravascular volume and may compromise placental perfusion.

3-17. The answer is c. (*Fauci, pp 1932-48.*) This patient has evidence for acute hepatitis as is suggested by the history, physical examination and laboratory data showing hepatocellular injury. The epidemiology favors acute hepatitis A; the patient's history of travel to Mexico and work as a teacher are risk factors for hepatitis A. The incubation period of about one month is also typical. Hepatitis B and C are less likely without evidence for drug abuse or blood transfusion. Antibody to hepatitis B surface antigen would not be evidence for acute hepatitis B. HCV RNA is the appropriate test for acute hepatitis C infection, but this disease typically causes mild transaminase elevation and rarely presents with icterus.. Liver biopsy is not indicated in acute hepatitis as the diagnosis is usually apparent from the examination, liver enzymes, and serological evidence of recent viral infection. Abdominal ultrasound would not be helpful as liver enzymes suggest hepatocellular damage, not biliary obstruction.

3-18. The answer is a. *(Brunicardi, pp 316-318.)* Specific exclusion criteria for liver transplantation are not formally established. Some of the more common contraindications to liver transplantation are ongoing or recent substance abuse, presence of active sepsis, current extrahepatic malignancy, poor cardiac or pulmonary function, and patients with hepatocellular carcinoma with metastatic disease, obvious vascular invasion, or significant tumor burden. Patients with hepatocellular carcinoma who would not tolerate resection because of portal hypertension and uncompensated liver disease can be successfully treated with liver transplantation. The best candidates are patients with a single lesion less than 5 cm in size or no more than three lesions, none of which are greater than 3 cm in size. The presence of hepatorenal syndrome is an indication, not a contraindication, to liver transplantation. Presence of an extrahepatic malignancy should defer transplantation for 2 years after curative therapy for their malignancy.

3-19. The answer is d. *(Ropper, pp 939-940.)* Motor neuron disease in the anterior horns of the spinal cord and damage to the corticospinal tracts or motor neurons contributing axons to the corticospinal tracts would account for these neurologic signs. Damage to the dorsal spinal root would be expected to produce sensory, rather than motor, deficits and would produce areflexia, rather than hyperreflexia, at the level of the injury. Damage to the ventral spinal roots would produce weakness and wasting, but no spasticity or hyperreflexia would develop. Purkinje cell damage would be expected to produce ataxia without substantial weakness. The arcuate fasciculus connects elements of the cerebral cortex not involved in the regulation of strength or motor tone.

3-20. The answer is b. *(Rosner, pp 43-67.)* Sensitivity is thought of as the probability that a symptom is present given that the person has the disease. In the above example, the "symptom" in question is a family history of breast cancer. Of women that have breast cancer, 5% have a family history; therefore the sensitivity of using family history as a predictor of breast cancer is 5%.

3-21. The answer is b. *(Kaplan, p 806.)* The essential feature of obsessive-compulsive personality disorder is a preoccupation with perfection, orderliness, and control. Individuals with this disorder lose the main point of an activity and miss deadlines because they pay too much attention to rules and details and are not satisfied with anything less than "perfection." As in other personality disorders, symptoms are ego-syntonic and create interpersonal, social, and occupational difficulties. Obsessive-compulsive disorder is differentiated from obsessive-compulsive personality disorder by the presence of obsessions and compulsions. In addition, patients with symptoms of obsessive-compulsive disorder view them as ego-dystonic. Patients with borderline personality disorder present with a history of pervasive instability of mood, relationships, and self-image beginning by early adulthood. Their behavior is often impulsive and self-damaging. Patients with bipolar disorder present with problems of mood stability; mood may be depressed for several weeks at a time, then euphoric. Patients with an anxiety disorder not otherwise specified present with anxiety as a main symptom, though they do not specifically fit any other, more specific anxiety disorder as per DSM-IV-TR (*Diagnostic and Statistical Manual* 4th ed, text revision).

3-22. The answer is b. *(Fauci, pp 241-242.)* Delayed gastric emptying (gastroparesis) is a common cause of recurrent vomiting, nausea, early satiety, and weight loss in poorly controlled diabetics. Abdominal discomfort is often nonspecific, but may be localized to the upper abdomen and often awakens the patient at night. Drugs with anticholinergic properties may aggravate the problem. The best diagnostic test is a scintigraphic gastric emptying study, which will show delay in gastric emptying. Treatment includes withdrawal of aggravating drugs such as opiates and those that have anticholinergic properties, good diabetes control, and drug therapy with metoclopropamide or erythromycin. The patient's symptoms are not those of esophageal disease (dysphagia, odynophagia), so a barium esophagram would not be useful. Her symptoms also do not suggest colonic pathology; in the absence of iron deficiency, colonoscopy would not be indicated. You would not order a liver biopsy in a patient with normal liver enzymes and CT scan of the abdomen. Small bowel biopsy would be indicated if her symptoms suggest intestinal malabsorption.

3-23. The answer is a. *(Rosen, p 1522.)* High clinical suspicion in this case is for **myasthenia gravis,** an autoimmune condition in which

acetylcholine receptor antibodies block acetylcholine binding and prevent normal neuromuscular conduction. The disease typically affects young women and older men and presents with **generalized weakness worsening with repetitive muscle use that is usually relieved with rest**. Ptosis and diplopia are usually present. The **edrophonium test** is used to help diagnose myasthenia gravis. It involves administering edrophonium, a short-acting anticholinesterase, which prevents acetylcholine breakdown. With the increased acetylcholine levels at the neuromuscular junction, the patient experiences a subjective and objective improvement of symptoms by preventing rapid breakdown of acetylcholine at the myoneural junction. Serologic testing **(b)** for antibodies to acetylcholine receptors is useful when positive and should be obtained in the workup of this patient. A negative test does not exclude the disorder. The electromyogram is diagnostic. **(c)** You may consider a CT scan to evaluate the patient for possible mass lesion or aneurysm that is causing her ptosis and diplopia. However, the clinical scenario is more consistent with myasthenia gravis. **(d)** An electrolyte panel will likely be normal. **(e)** If the edrophonium test is normal, a lumbar puncture should be considered.

3-24. The answer is b. (*Cunningham, pp 1130-1131, 1276-1293, 1307-1310.*) Early-onset group B streptococcus disease occurs within 1 week of birth. Signs of the disease include respiratory distress, apnea, and shock. Late-onset disease usually occurs after 7 days and manifests as meningitis. Listeriosis during pregnancy can be asymptomatic or cause a febrile illness that is confused with influenza, pyelonephritis, or meningitis. *L. monocytogenes,* the causative bacteria is usually acquired through food-borne transmission from manure-contaminated cabbage, pasteurized milk, and fresh Mexican-style cheeses. Fetal infection is characterized by granulomatous lesions with microabscesses. Early onset neonatal sepsis is a common manifestation of listeriosis during pregnancy, and late onset listeriosis occurs after 3 to 4 weeks as meningitis, which is similar to group B streptococci. However, listeriosis infection is much less common.

3-25. The answer is d. (*Fauci, pp 541-545.*) The lesion has characteristics of melanoma (Remember the ABCDs: *a*symmetry, irregular or ill-defined *b*order, dark black or variegated *c*olor, and *d*iameter greater than 6 mm). A full-thickness excisional biopsy is required for diagnosis and should not be delayed. Shave biopsy of a suspected melanoma is always contraindicated. Diagnosis is urgent; the lesion cannot be observed over time. Once the diagnosis of melanoma is made, the tumor must then be staged to determine prognosis and treatment.

3-26. The answer is e. (*South-Paul, pp 549-557.*) When discussing CAM, physicians should help patients make informed choices. Many practices, including acupuncture, biofeedback, homeopathy, and meditation are low risk if used by competent practitioners. Many herbal substances can interact with traditional medications and cause harm. St. John's wort can cause serotonin syndrome when used with a selective serotonin reuptake inhibitor like paroxetine. Megavitamins carry with them the risk of toxicity. Special diets, including the macrobiotic diet (high complex carbohydrate, low-fat, vegetarian diet) may have harmful effects, including undesirable changes in weight and bowel habits. Ginkgo biloba has antiplatelet effects, and may cause bleeding when taken with aspirin.

3-27 to 3-31. The answers are 27-c, 28-b, 29-d, 30-e, 31-a. (*Hay, pp 339-340, 350-351, 357. Kliegman, pp 341 345, 354-355, 2913-2918. McMillan, pp 210, 752-764, 767-772. Rudolph, pp 360, 368-371, 373-376.*) The most important aspect of the management of lead poisoning is the identification and withdrawal of the source of the lead. Patients with symptomatic lead poisoning or extremely high lead levels in the blood (> 70 µg/dL) should be treated with both dimercaprol and calcium EDTA. With milder poisoning, intravenous or intramuscular calcium EDTA or, more likely, oral dimercaptosuccinic acid can be used.

N-acetylcysteine (NAC) is an effective treatment for acetaminophen poisoning and acts by removing hepatotoxic metabolites. It should be given within 16 hours of ingestion; after 36 hours it is probably ineffective.

Morphine and other narcotics used in the labor and delivery process produce their major toxic effect by suppression of ventilation. Ventilatory support can be necessary initially, but naloxone is a specific antidote and can be very rapidly effective. The effect of naloxone can wear off more quickly than the effects of the drug for which it was given, so careful observation and repeated doses may be necessary.

Salicylate poisoning produces metabolic acidosis and respiratory alkalosis (although this latter feature is often missed in young children), hyperglycemia or hypoglycemia, paradoxical aciduria, dehydration, and lethargy. Excretion of salicylates in the urine can be markedly enhanced by the administration of acetazolamide and IV sodium bicarbonate. Hemodialysis can also be used.

Organophosphate insecticides are absorbed from all sites and act by inhibiting cholinesterases, thereby leading to the accumulation of high levels of acetylcholine. This affects the parasympathetic nervous system, muscle, and the CNS. Treatment of a patient contaminated with organophosphate insecticide will include thorough washing of the pesticide from the skin, inducing emesis or performing gastric lavage, supporting ventilation, and administering atropine followed by pralidoxime (2-PAM).

3-32. The answer is a. *(Townsend, pp 1802-1812.)* CABG is indicated in patients with angina (chronic, unstable, or postinfarction) and in asymptomatic patients with ischemia on cardiac stress tests. Operative mortality depends on the presence of risk factors such as age, other comorbidities, and preoperative ventricular function. Mortality in low risk, younger patients is approximately 3%. CABG offers a long-term survival benefit in patients with multivessel disease, left main coronary artery disease, and one-vessel and two-vessel disease with proximal left anterior descending coronary artery obstruction. CABG is the treatment of choice in diabetic patients. CABG is not indicated for patients with congestive heart failure unless this condition is ischemic in origin and angiography identifies disease amenable to surgical revascularization.

3-33. The answer is b. *(Kaplan, p 911.)* Alcohol intoxication and an overt stressor (impending breakup with the girlfriend) are both predictors of violence. Demographically, males from the ages of 15 to 24 are more likely to commit violent acts, and this patient is outside that age range. Also, those with low socioeconomic statuses and few social supports are more likely to commit violent acts. While verbal threats of physical violence do increase the risk of subsequent physical violence, the age difference of the couple in question has no bearing on the prediction of violence.

3-34. The answer is e. *(Rosen, pp 2643-2644.)* **Inhalation anthrax** is a rare, but life-threatening disease, with mortality rates exceeding 90%. It is caused by inhaling *B anthracis* spores into the lungs. Initially, the patient develops flu-like symptoms. Within 24 to 48 hours, the clinical course may abruptly deteriorate to septic shock, respiratory failure, and mediastinitis. Chest x-ray may reveal a widened mediastinum. Death usually results within 3 days. Anthrax is normally a disease of sheep, cattle, and horses. As there is no evidence for human-to-human transmission, disease in humans occurs when spores are inhaled. Working with untreated animal hides increases the risk for anthrax exposure.

Though *S pneumoniae* and *H influenzae* (**a and d**) can cause respiratory failure, it is unlikely to occur in a healthy 32-year-old man. (**b**) Diphtheria is a potentially life-threatening disease that is characterized by a gray-green pseudomembrane covering the tonsils and pharyngeal mucosa. *Coxiella* *burnetii* (**c**) is the organism that causes Q fever. It is similar to *B anthracis* in that sheep, cattle, and goats are the primary reservoirs. However, deterioration because of Q fever is not as rapid as that seen in anthrax.

3-35. The answer is b. (*Mengel, pp 300-306.*) Hypertrophic cardiomyopathy can be associated with atrial fibrillation or ventricular tachycardia. The characteristic heart murmur associated with it is a systolic ejection murmur (like aortic stenosis) worsening with Valsalva maneuver. Mitral valve prolapse would have a different characteristic murmur. Dilated cardiomyopathy and CHF would likely be associated with other symptoms. Atrial fibrillation would not be associated with a regular rhythm.

3-36. The answer is d. (*Kaplan p 710.*) In transvestic fetishism, patients, usually heterosexual males, experience recurrent and intense sexual arousal while they are cross-dressing. Masturbation, with fantasies of sexual attractiveness while dressed as a woman, usually accompanies the cross-dressing. Wearing an article of women's clothing or dressing as a woman while having intercourse can also be sexually exciting for these patients. The condition often begins in childhood or early adolescence. Males with this disorder consider themselves to be male, but some have gender dysphoria. For diagnostic purposes, the behavior must persist over a period of at least 6 months.

3-37. The answer is a. (*Brunicardi, pp 742-744.*) The patient has a mycotic aortic aneurysm, which is a sequela of infection, most commonly with either *Staphylococcus* or *Salmonella*. Treatment for infrarenal mycotic aortic aneurysms has traditionally been that an axillofemoral bypass is performed and then the involved intra-abdominal aorta is excised. If the aorta is debrided and replaced, autogenous graft material is used (eg, superficial femoral vein). Antibiotic therapy is also administered for 3 to 6 months.

3-38. The answer is d. (*Stenchever, pp 889-898.*) By definition, an IVP showing hydronephrosis would mean the cancer has extended to the pelvic side wall and thus a stage III carcinoma, specifically stage IIIb. Such staging applies even if there is no palpable tumor beyond the cervix. IVP, cystoscopy, and proctosigmoidoscopy are diagnostic tests used to stage cervical cancer along with pelvic examination. However, it is important to understand that while the results of only certain tests are used to stage cervical cancer, this does not limit the physician from performing other diagnostic tests (such as CT scans of the abdomen, pelvis, or chest) that in his or her judgment are required for appropriate medical care and decision making.

3-39. The answer is a. (*South-Paul, pp 329-342.*) Iron deficiency may be asymptomatic, but patients may present with varying degrees of weakness, fatigue, dizziness, palpitations, or exercise intolerance. On physical examination, one may see pallor and tachycardia. Pica, the craving of ice, clay, or other substances is particularly associated with iron deficiency. Lead, anemia of chronic disease, vitamin B$_{12}$, and folate deficiency usually do not cause pica.

3-40. The answer is n. (*Ropper, pp 644-646.*) This woman is at relatively high risk for AIDS encephalopathy because she has required transfusion of clotting factors that have until recently been available only from pooled samples of blood products. The neurologic deficits that she exhibits are not specific for HIV-1–associated subacute encephalomyelitis (AIDS encephalitis) and are quite compatible with multiple sclerosis (MS). That her MRI does not reveal plaques of demyelination scattered throughout the brain makes the diagnosis of MS improbable. To establish the diagnosis of AIDS encephalopathy, HIV-1 antibodies should be sought and the helper/suppressor (CD4/CD8) T-lymphocyte ratio should be checked. Patients with symptomatic AIDS usually have a CD4/CD8 T-lymphocyte ratio of less than 0.5.

3-41. The answer is o. (*Ropper, pp 345-346.*) Obesity associated with hypersomnia qualifies as pickwickian syndrome if the patient exhibits other characteristic features, such as sleep apnea. The patient with this syndrome is likely to have hypoxemia and pulmonary hypertension. Smoking increases the risk of developing the syndrome. Sleep attacks usually abate with cessation of smoking and weight loss.

3-42. The answer is e. (*Ropper, pp 638-640.*) With herpes encephalitis in the person who is not immunodeficient, the first clinical signs of disease are likely to be psychiatric. Depression, irritability, and labile affect are especially common. The organic basis for the encephalopathy usually becomes self-evident when the affected person has a seizure. Because the temporal lobe is especially involved by herpes encephalitis, the initial seizure is likely to be complex partial, but seizures often become more generalized. EEG will usually reveal the focal character of the cerebral damage. Intracranial pressure is usually increased with a fulminant infection. Temporal lobe swelling may be severe enough to produce lethal herniation.

3-43. The answer is i. (*Ropper, pp 771-790.*) Optic neuritis is often the first symptom that motivates the patient with multiple sclerosis to consult a physician. Clumsiness, stumbling, and other symptoms of ataxia are usually dismissed as inconsequential by the patient. Even those with profoundly slow and slurred speech are often unaware of their dysarthria. When the patient finally does consult a physician, multiple neurologic abnormalities are usually evident. This patient would be expected to have a positive swinging flashlight test (Marcus Gunn pupil) and evidence of widespread demyelination on MRI of the head.

3-44. The answer is l. *(Ropper, p 596.)* With acute bacterial meningitis, the time between the first symptoms and death may be only days. A petechial rash developing over the lower parts of the body in the setting of fever, headache, nuchal rigidity, photophobia, and stupor must be considered presumptive evidence of a meningococcal meningitis. Rapid diagnosis and treatment is essential if the patient is to survive. The spinal fluid typically reveals a low glucose content, high protein content, and leukocytosis with a large number of polymorphonuclear cells. Treatment with intravenous penicillin G, 12 million to 15 million U daily (divided into four to six doses) early in the course of illness may decide whether the patient survives more than a few hours or days.

3-45. The answer is a. *(Ropper, p 287.)* After significant head trauma, the victim is at considerable risk for a seizure. A patient's seizure threshold is lowest when he or she is asleep or sleep-deprived. If the posttraumatic seizure occurs during sleep, it may go unnoticed. The patient's improving cognition suggests a postictal state. His hemiparesis is probably a Todd paralysis, but any patient with posttraumatic seizures and focal weakness must be investigated for an acute or chronic subdural hematoma.

3-46. The answer is j. *(Ropper, pp 967-969.)* Carbon tetrachloride is a potent hepatic toxin. This woman may have attempted to commit suicide by drinking cleaning fluid. As hepatic damage progressed, she developed fetor hepaticus, a distinctive smell to her breath that reflects a profound metabolic disturbance. The serum ammonia level rose as liver function declined. The triphasic waves typically seen in hepatic encephalopathy may occur with uremia and other causes of metabolic encephalopathy.

Block 4

Answers

4-1. The answer is d. *(Rosen, pp 226-231.)* This patient has a significant risk factor for having an **ectopic pregnancy**. Tubal ligations raise the likelihood of having an ectopic pregnancy by providing an outlet for improper implantation of an embryo into the abdominal cavity or somewhere outside of the uterus. Implantation most commonly occurs in the fallopian tubes, 95% of the time. Again, a β-hCG is crucial in the beginning stages in the workup of this patient. In a normal pregnancy, the β-hCG doubles every 2 days and typically only increases by two-thirds in ectopic pregnancies. Progesterone levels also differ and may be helpful. A transvaginal ultrasound is also warranted to determine the size and location of the ectopic and any associated free fluid indicating rupture. β-hCG levels dictate whether a transvaginal (> 1500 mIU/mL) or transabdominal (> 6500 mIU/mL) approach should be used. Smaller, nonruptured ectopics may be treated with methotrexate. However, this patient is hemodynamically compromised and has most likely ruptured. Surgical intervention is warranted in these cases. Patients with ectopic pregnancies may also present with back or flank pain, syncope or peritonitis in cases with significant abdominal hemorrhage. Risk factors also include previous ectopics, intrauterine devices, PID, sexually transmitted diseases (STDs), in vitro fertilization, and recent elective abortion. The incidence of a coexisting heterotopic pregnancy is about 1/30,000 but increases to 1/8000 in women on fertility drugs.

Both gastrointestinal (GI) and gynecological conditions should be included in the differential diagnosis of women presenting with abdominal pain, and appendicitis (**a**) is often at the top of the list. However, its probability is lowered by the associated vaginal bleeding. PID (**b**) often presents with gradual pelvic pain and discharge with other systemic signs of an infectious etiology, such as fever. Placenta previa (**c**) usually presents with **painless** vaginal bleeding in the second trimester. Abruptio placentae (**e**) also presents in the second or third trimester and is **painful**.

4-2. The answer is c. *(Rosner, pp 43-67.)* A false-negative is defined as a person who tests negative, but who is actually positive. In the above example,

2% of the positive people test negative. Therefore, the false-negative rate is 2% in this case. Sensitivity is defined as the probability that the test would be positive, given that the person has strep throat. The specificity is the probability that the test would be negative if the person does *not* have strep. The false-positive rate is defined as the percent of people who test positive, but are actually negative. The positive predictive value is the probability that a person has an illness, given that the test is positive.

4-3. The answer is c. (*Fauci pp 2380*) Hypercalcemia must first be confirmed since misleading laboratory values can be caused by hemoconcentration of the serum sample. Ninety percent of hypercalcemia is attributed either to hyperparathyroidism or to malignancy. Almost all patients with malignancy-associated hypercalcemia have previously diagnosed cancer or symptoms (weight loss, anorexia, cough, hemoptysis) to suggest this diagnosis. In this otherwise healthy patient, confirmed hypercalcemia should lead to measurement of intact parathyroid hormone (iPTH). Other causes of hypercalcemia include familial hypocalciuric hypercalcemia, Vitamin D intoxication, sarcoidosis and other granulomatous diseases, hyperthyroidism, prolonged immobilization, and milk-alkali syndrome. Thyroid studies and liver enzymes (to evaluate for granulomatous hepatitis) might be ordered if the iPTH level is suppressed. Urine calcium excretion is assessed before parathyroidectomy to rule out familial hypocalciuric hypercalcemia, which can otherwise mimic hyperparathyroidism. Urine calcium determination, however, would not be the first test obtained in the assessment of hypercalcemia. Osteoporosis should be considered in this postmenopausal woman with hyperparathyroidism and appropriate screening for osteoporosis performed with central dual x-ray absorptiometry (DXA).

4-4. The answer is c. (*Ropper, pp 593-601.*) The immediate concern is that the patient has bacterial meningitis, and she should be treated. A lumbar puncture and blood drawn to obtain cultures should be done; however, it can take a few days for the results to come back, and it may be too late for the patient by then. Oral azithromycin is not the proper treatment for bacterial meningitis. Intravenous acyclovir would be used to treat herpes encephalitis.

4-5. The answer is d. (*Hay, pp 163-174. Kliegman, pp 127-130. McMillan, pp 655-661. Rudolph, pp 231-233.*) The young lady in the question could have any number of problems, and all of the answers could ultimately prove to be helpful. As a first step, however, a close look at her weight in comparison to previous ones is in order; she has some physical examination findings seen with bulimia (dental decay, irritated uvula), and others seen with anorexia nervosa (lanugo, thinning hair, low resting heart rate, hypothermia, secondary amenorrhea).

Eating disorders have become increasingly prevalent in recent years. Symptoms of finicky appetite, progressively restricted food intake, distress at looking fat, and compulsively pursuing thinness can appear after puberty. Parents may not appreciate the magnitude of weight loss until it reaches 10% or more of body weight, because those girls will not undress in their parents' presence and because the facial contours are the last parts to be affected. Bulimia usually appears in mid adolescence rather than early adolescence and is characterized by sessions of gorging, often in secret and often involving a single favored snack food such as ice cream, cake, or candy, although it may also be manifested as immoderate eating at mealtimes. This gorging is followed by secret bouts of self-induced vomiting. Some bulimics also use laxatives and purgatives. Physical consequences of bulimia include esophageal varices and hemorrhage; dental decay, especially of anterior teeth (because of exposure of enamel to gastric HCl); and a swollen, reddened, irritated uvula (also from chronic HCl exposure). Physical consequences of anorexia include profound weight loss (25%-30% or more of body weight), dehydration, facial and arm hirsutism, loss of hair of the head, bradycardia, cardiac conduction problems, reduced cardiac output, hypothermia, impaired renal function, multiple malnutrition effects (including avitaminoses), a primary or secondary amenorrhea, and osteoporosis. Significant mortality in treatment-resistant cases is seen. The psychologic component of these disorders is not a unitary one. Some anorexic patients have an underlying obsessive-compulsive or narcissistic personality disorder, some are borderline psychotic, and some are depressed. Bulimic patients have a significant underlying depression. Patients with eating disorders have exceedingly ambivalent feelings toward parents, especially mothers, and in turn evoke great ambivalence on the part of parents. Therapy includes behavior modification to deal with eating behavior per se, family therapy, and individual or group therapy. Imipramine, when used appropriately, is a useful adjunct treatment for this condition. In cases of life-threatening degrees of weight loss or vomiting, hospitalization to limit freedom, restore physiologic equilibrium, and provide a controlled eating environment can be indicated.

4-6. The answer is c. (*South-Paul, pp 558-565.*) The World Health Organization published guidelines for pain control in 1996. These guidelines have been well-studied and lead to effective pain control in most situations. In general, failing nonopioid pain control should lead to the use of opioid analgesics. Steroids have limited, if any, use in chronic cancer pain. Fentanyl patches, even at the lowest dose, may be excessive in opiate naïve patients, and should never be used alone. Most start with immediate-release morphine sulfate to determine a baseline need. This can be converted to sustained release quickly, and titrated based on pain control. Patient-controlled analgesia devices have an important role, but require intravenous or subcutaneous administration, and should not be used first-line, unless pain is extreme.

4-7. The answer is d. (*DiSaia, pp 55-62.*) The main routes of spread of cervical cancer include vaginal mucosa, myometrium, paracervical lymphatics, and direct extension into the parametrium. The prevalence of lymph node disease correlates with the stage of malignancy. Primary node groups involved in the spread of cervical cancer include the paracervical, parametrial, obturator, hypogastric, external iliac, and sacral nodes, essentially in that order. Less commonly, there is involvement in the common iliac, inguinal, and para-aortic nodes. In stage I, the pelvic nodes are positive in approximately 15% of cases and the para-aortic nodes in 6%. In stage II, pelvic nodes are positive in 28% of cases and para-aortic nodes in 16%. In stage III, pelvic nodes are positive in 47% of cases and para-aortic nodes in 28%.

4-8. The answer is c. (*Heys, pp 614-623.*) Malignant tumors require energy substrates to grow and ordinarily claim these substrates from the host. In animal studies, withholding dietary proteins diminishes the rate of tumor growth. There is no evidence in the human to suggest acceleration of tumor growth when nutritional support is provided. There is also no evidence that nutritional therapy improves the response of the tumor to therapy. For nearly a century, the association of stomach cancer and diet has been recognized. Among the wide variety of substances incriminated are nitrates and nitrosamides in food and drinking water. There is evidence that regular ingestion of vitamin C from childhood may reduce the formation of carcinogens, though reduction in the incidence of cancer has not been demonstrated. Excess amounts of dietary fat and deficiency of fiber have been clearly associated with colon cancer. Animal fats have also been associated with cancer of the exocrine pancreas, the prostate, and the endometrium. Alcohol consumption, especially when combined with cigarette smoking, increases the incidence of esophageal cancer. Consumption of alcohol also increases the incidence of pancreatitis, but not pancreatic cancer.

4-9. The answer is c. (*Fauci, pp 573-575.*) It is likely that most colon cancers start out as adenomatous polyps; this explains the rationale for using colonoscopy as a preventative test for colon cancer, despite the fact that proof is lacking. Larger polyps, sessile polyps, and those that contain villous elements are more likely to harbor malignancies. Patients who have had one adenomatous polyp removed have a 30% to 50% chance of developing another polyp, but the regrowth is slow (taking at least 3 years to become clinically significant). Repeat colonoscopy is, therefore, recommended 3 years after the adenoma has been removed.

4-10. The answer is e. *(Kaplan, p 918.)* Discontinuation of the antipsychotic medication or a dosage decrease are the initial interventions recommended when tardive dyskinesia is first diagnosed. If discontinuation is not possible and dosage decrease is not effective, clozapine has been proven effective in ameliorating and suppressing the symptoms of tardive dyskinesia.

4-11. The answer is a. *(Ropper, p 1221.)* Men with myotonic dystrophy characteristically exhibit problems with relaxing their grip, hypersomnolence, premature baldness, testicular atrophy, and cataracts. The EMG pattern displayed by these patients is often referred to as the *dive bomber pattern* because of the characteristic sound produced when the evoked action potentials are heard. The cardiac defect that evolves in these persons usually requires pacemaker implantation to avoid sudden death. Psychiatric problems also develop in many patients with myotonic dystrophy, but their basis is unknown.

4-12. The answer is d. *(Hay, pp 125-126. Kliegman, pp 2385-2386. McMillan, pp 558-559. Rudolph, p 248.)* Gynecomastia is a common occurrence in adolescent boys, especially during Tanner stage 2 or 3. It can occur unilaterally or bilaterally, and can affect one breast more significantly than the other. It is thought to be caused by a temporary reduction in the testosterone to estradiol ratio. Spontaneous regression usually occurs; it rarely lasts for more than 2 years. In the child who otherwise has a normal physical examination and no significant past medical history, reassurance of the benign nature of the condition is all that is required for most cases. Rarely, the gynecomastia is significant; antiestrogen agents can be utilized or surgery can be considered. Other, more serious causes for this condition include Klinefelter syndrome, hyperthyroidism, hormone-producing tumors, and drugs (including marijuana). A thorough history and physical examination can help eliminate these relatively unusual causes.

4-13. The answer is a. *(Rosen, pp 788-793.)* Only two venomous lizards are found in the world, both of which whose natural habitat is in the southwestern United States and Mexico. These animals are usually not aggressive, despite the Gila monster's name, and bites are usually a result of direct handling as in this case. Both the Gila monster and the Mexican-beaded lizard are easily identified by their thick bodies, beaded scales with either white and black or pink and black configuration. Envenomation from these bites occurs from the glands along the lower jaw and introduced into the victim through grooved teeth, which the animal uses to continuously chew after it has bitten down. These teeth may become embedded in the victim, thereby distributing more venom.

Antivenin (**b**) is not available for these bites, as they are rarely fatal. Broad-spectrum antibiotics (**d**) and tetanus prophylaxis (**c**) should be administered at a later interval. Applying a suction device (**e**) as in snakebites is not warranted. The patient should be observed for at least 6 hours for systemic effects.

4-14. The answer is a. (*Rodeck, pp 851-853.*) Toxoplasmosis, a protozoal infection caused by *T. gondii*, can result from ingestion of raw or undercooked meat infected by the organism or from contact with infected cat feces. The French, because their diet includes raw meat, have a high incidence. The incidence of toxoplasmosis in pregnant women is estimated to be 1 in every 150 to 700 pregnancies. Infection early in pregnancy may cause abortion; later in pregnancy, the fetus may become infected. A small number of infected infants develop involvement of the central nervous system or the eye; most infants who have the disease, however, escape serious clinical problems.

4-15. The answer is a. (*Fauci, p 192.*) The fact that vision is preserved excludes optic neuritis and cavernous sinus thrombosis. Optic neuritis will produce pain in the affected eye and may be associated with a normal optic disc, but visual acuity should be deficient and an afferent pupillary defect should be apparent. Cavernous sinus thrombosis usually produces proptosis and pain, but impaired venous drainage from the eye should interfere with acuity, and the retina should appear profoundly disturbed. With a diphtheritic polyneuropathy, an ophthalmoplegia may develop, but this would not be limited to one eye and is not usually associated with facial trauma. Transverse sinus thrombosis may produce cerebrocortical dysfunction or stroke, but ophthalmoplegia would not be a manifestation of this problem. The history and examination findings are classic for a superficial infection developing into orbital cellulitis.

4-16. The answer is a. (*South-Paul, pp 310-328. McPhee, pp 604-607.*) The patient described in this question has pancreatitis. Gallstones cause the majority of cases of pancreatitis. Alcohol causes about 30% of the cases.

Ten to thirty percent are idiopathic. Less common causes include hypercalcemia, hyperlipidemia, abdominal trauma, medications, infections, and instrumentation (for instance, after an ERCP).

4-17. The answer is c. *(Townsend, pp 2098-2102.)* The patient's history of the "worst headache of her life" and initial examination findings are highly suggestive of a subarachnoid hemorrhage. A CT scan without contrast will show a localized clot, diffusely distributed hemorrhage, intraventricular hemorrhage, or intraparenchymal hemorrhage 80% to 90% of the time. If the CT scan is negative, and the history and physical examination strongly support a subarachnoid hemorrhage, then a lumbar puncture is obtained. As opposed to traumatic lumbar taps, the red blood cell count does not diminish between the first and last tubes collected when a subarachnoid hemorrhage is present. Xanthochromia is the yellow appearance of cerebrospinal fluid caused by the degradation of heme to bilirubin in the red blood cells entering the CSF during the bleeding. Workup should then proceed to a four-vessel cerebral angiogram to assess for a cerebral aneurysm. Given that only about 85% of cerebral aneurysms are identified on the initial study, a second angiogram should be performed within 7 to 10 days after the first study to completely rule out an aneurysm. Initial management consists of medical therapy to counteract vasospasm, blood pressure control, and anticonvulsant therapy. Although hydrocephalus can result from blockage of the arachnoidal channels, ventriculostomy is not the surgical management of choice. Surgical treatment should be initiated early and consists of craniotomy with clipping of the aneurysm.

4-18. The answer is c. *(Rosen, pp 1549-1583.)* **Steroid psychosis** is described as a constellation of psychiatric symptoms within the first 5 days of treatment with a corticosteroid. Studies indicate that the amount needed to produce this effect is greater than 40 mg of prednisone, or its equivalent, prescribed daily. Symptoms include emotional lability, anxiety, distractibility, pressured speech, sensory flooding, insomnia, depression, agitation, auditory and visual hallucinations, intermittent memory impairment, mutism, disturbances of body image, and delusions and hypomania. It is important to note that previous history of psychologic difficulties does not predict the development of steroid psychosis. Symptoms can be very severe and should be taken into account when prescribing this medication to patients. Three percent of patients with steroid psychosis commit suicide.

The most common side effect of β-blockers (**a**) is a depressed mood, owing to its sympatholytic effects; however, these are generally mild and do not require treatment. Oral contraceptives (**b**), although hormonal in nature, are not thought to produce psychiatric symptoms. Calcium-channel blockers (**e**) and NSAIDs (**d**) have not shown to cause psychosis.

4-19. The answer is a. (*Fauci, pp 1577-1579.*) In all patients in whom primary pulmonary hypertension is confirmed, acute drug testing with a pulmonary vasodilator is necessary to assess the extent of pulmonary vascular reactivity. Inhaled nitric oxide, intravenous adenosine, and intravenous prostacyclin have all been used. Patients who have a good response to the short-acting vasodilator are tried on a long-acting calcium channel antagonist under direct hemodynamic monitoring. Prostacyclin given via the pulmonary artery through a right heart catheter has been approved for patients who are functional class III or IV and have not responded to calcium channel antagonists. Sildenafil (a selective phosphodiesterase-5 inhibitor), treprostinil (a prostacyclin) and bosentan (an endothelin receptor antagonist) have also recently been approved for class III and IV disease. These drugs are not usually used empirically. Lung transplantation is reserved for late stages of the disease when patients are unresponsive to prostacyclin. The disease does not appear to recur after transplantation.

4-20. The answer is b. (*Hay, pp 927-928. Kliegman, pp 890-891. McMillan, pp 2467-2468. Rudolph, p 799.*) The patient described has Wiskott-Aldrich syndrome, an X-linked recessive combined immunodeficiency characterized by thrombocytopenia, eczema, and increased susceptibility to infection. Problems occur early, and frequently prolonged bleeding from the circumcision site is the first clue. The thrombocytopenia also manifests as bloody diarrhea and easy bruising. Patients have impaired humoral immunity with a low serum IgM and a normal or slightly low IgG; they also have cellular immunity problems, with decreased T cells and depressed lymphocyte response. Few live past their teens, frequently succumbing to malignancy caused by EBV infection.

Idiopathic thrombocytopenic purpura (ITP) is an isolated and usually transient thrombocytopenia thought to be secondary to a viral infection. These children do not have increased susceptibility to infection. Acute lymphocytic leukemia (ALL) usually presents with abnormalities in all three cell lines, and does not have a prolonged course as in the described patient. Adenosine deaminase (ADA) deficiency is a type of severe combined immunodeficiency (SCID) but patients always have lymphopenia from birth; platelets are not affected. Partial thymic hypoplasia (partial DiGeorge) patients usually do not have problems early on and can grow up normally, and they do not have thrombocytopenia.

4-21. The answer is d. (*Kandel, p 865.*) Huntington disease is transmitted in an autosomal dominant fashion. The age at which the patient becomes symptomatic is variable and has no effect on the probability of transmitting the disease. The defect underlying this degenerative disease is an abnormal expansion of a region of chromosome 4 containing a triplicate repeat (CAG) sequence. Normal individuals have between 6 and 34 copies of this CAG section; patients with Huntington disease may have from 37 to more than 100 repeats. Once expanded beyond 40 copies, the repeats are unstable and may further increase as they are passed on from one generation to the next. An increased number of repeats leads to a phenomenon known as *anticipation,* by which successive generations have earlier disease onset.

4-22. The answer is e. (*Rakel, pp 639-643.*) The condition described is a thrombosed external hemorrhoid. External hemorrhoids are defined as hemorrhoids arising distal to the dentate line. When they thrombose, they are associated with acute pain and are hard and nodular on physical examination. The excision can be safely done in the office with local anesthesia. It eliminates pain immediately and eliminates the risk of reoccurrence. Hydrocortisone would not be helpful. Rubber band ligation and sclerotherapy should be reserved for internal hemorrhoids. Incision and drainage of the hemorrhoid increases the risk of reoccurrence and can lead to infection of the retained clot.

4-23. The answer is b. (*Ropper, pp 931-934.*) More than 10% of patients with Friedreich disease develop diabetes mellitus. A more life-threatening complication of this degenerative disease is the disturbance of the cardiac conduction system that often develops. Visual problems occur with the hyperglycemia of uncontrolled diabetes mellitus, but even Friedreich patients without diabetes develop optic atrophy late in the course of the degenerative disease.

4-24. The answer is e. (*Moore and Jefferson, pp 11, 165-167.*) A social phobia is a persistent and overwhelming fear of humiliation or embarrassment in social or performance situations. This leads to high levels of distress and avoidance of those situations. Often, physical symptoms of anxiety such as blushing, trembling, sweating, or tachycardia are triggered when the patient feels under evaluation or scrutiny.

4-25. The answer is a. (*Brunicardi, pp 1501-1504.*) In most children, umbilical hernias close spontaneously by the age of 4 and need not be repaired unless incarcerated or symptomatic. Omphalocele and gastroschisis result in evisceration of bowel and require emergency surgical treatment to effect immediate or staged reduction and abdominal wall closure. Patent urachal or omphalomesenteric ducts result from incomplete closure of embryonic connections from the bladder and ileum, respectively, to the abdominal wall. They are appropriately treated by excision of the tracts and closure of the bladder or ileum.

4-26. The answer is c. (*Mengel, pp 396-400.*) When a patient presents with acute shortness of breath and an increased respiratory rate, PE must be ruled out. The patient in this case is taking oral contraceptives, increasing her risk for PE. After appropriate workup, anticoagulation should be initiated. An allergic reaction, asthma or bronchitis would likely cause an abnormal lung examination.

4-27. The answer is d. (*Fauci, pp 1565-1566.*) This patient's presentation strongly suggests aortic dissection. Aortic insufficiency is common with proximal dissection, as is hypertension and evidence of CHF. Hypotension may be present in severe cases. Distal dissection can lead to obstruction of other major arteries with neurological symptoms (carotids), bowel ischemia, or renal compromise. In aortic dissection, the first line of defense is emergent therapy with parenteral beta-blockers. After beta-blockade is established, nitroprusside is commonly used to titrate systolic blood pressure to less than 120. The diagnosis is established with transesophageal echo, MR, or CT angiography. Urgent surgery may be required, especially in proximal (Type A) dissections.

Although endocarditis may cause aortic insufficiency, this patient's sudden onset of symptoms as well as widened mediastinum would be unusual in endocarditis. Myocardial ischemia can cause mitral (but not aortic) insufficiency. Furosemide might help the pulmonary edema but would not address the primary problem; digoxin increases shear force on the aortic wall and could worsen the dissection. Anticoagulation is contraindicated if aortic dissection is suspected, as it may increase the risk of fatal rupture and exsanguinating hemorrhage.

4-28. The answer is d. (*Hay, pp 772-776, 1040. Kliegman, pp 2544-2547. McMillan, p 2325. Rudolph, pp 2293-2294, 2406.*) The child in the question appears to have myotonic muscular dystrophy. An elevated creatine kinase (especially in the preclinical phase) often is found, and psychomotor retardation can be the presenting complaint (but may be identified only in retrospect). Ptosis, baldness, hypogonadism, facial immobility with distal muscle wasting (in older children), and neonatal respiratory distress (in the newborn period) are major features of this disorder. Cataracts are commonly seen, presenting either congenitally or at any point during childhood. The prominence of distal muscle weakness in this disease is in contrast to the proximal muscle weakness seen in most other forms of myopathies. The diagnosis is confirmed by identifying typical findings on muscle biopsy. Seizures are not a feature of myotonic dystrophy. Enlarged gonads are associated with fragile X syndrome, and hirsutism is found (among other things) in children with congenital adrenal hyperplasia.

4-29. The answer is e. *(South-Paul, pp 641-646.)* Adherence is a complex issue for physicians and patients. In patients who do not adhere to their doctors' advice, the reasons usually relate to the patients' beliefs, goals and expectations. Asking the patient if he takes his medications is unlikely to yield accurate information, as the answer to this question is often an automatic "yes." However, patients will give accurate information about adherence about 80% of the time if the physician asks well-framed questions. By asking specific questions about names, dosages, and times, the physician will be more likely to elicit information about compliance. Another tactic may be to give permission for admitting noncompliance by saying something like, "Some of my patients find it difficult to remember to take their medications. Does this ever happen to you?"

Performing pill counts, measuring serum blood levels, and evaluating outcomes have not been shown in the medical literature to be effective measures of compliance.

4-30. The answer is a. *(Fauci p. 801.)* The striking features of this infection are its rapid onset and progression to a cellulitis characterized by dusky dark red erythema, bullae formation, and anesthesia over the area. These are clues to necrotizing fasciitis, a rapidly spreading deep soft tissue infection. The organism, usually *S pyogenes*, reaches the deep fascia from the site of penetrating trauma. Prompt surgical exploration down to fascia or muscle may be lifesaving. Necrotic tissue is Gram stained and cultured—streptococci, staphylococci, mixed anaerobic infection, or clostridia are all possible pathogens. Antibiotics to cover these organisms are important but not as important as prompt surgical debridement. Acute osteomyelitis is considered when cellulitis does not respond to antibiotic therapy, but would not present with this rapidity.

4-31. The answer is c. *(Cunningham, pp 92, 96, 208, 212, 390-392, 882.)* Measurement of the fetal crown-rump length is the most accurate means of estimating gestational age. In the first trimester, this ultrasound measurement is accurate to within 3 to 5 days. Estimating the uterine size on physical examination can result in an error of 1 to 2 weeks in the first trimester. Quantification of serum HCG cannot be used to determine gestational age, because at any gestational age the HCG number can vary widely in normal pregnancies. A single serum progesterone level cannot be used to date a pregnancy; however, it can be used to establish that an early pregnancy is developing normally. Serum progesterone levels less than 5 ng/mL usually indicate a nonviable pregnancy, while levels greater than 25 ng/mL indicate a normal intrauterine pregnancy. Progesterone levels in conjunction with quantitative HCG levels are often used to determine the presence of an ectopic pregnancy.

4-32. The answer is d. (*Fleischer and Ludwig, pp 834-835.*) This is a case of **erythema infectiosum** or **Fifth disease**. Infection by **parvovirus B19** produces this pattern of a **"slapped cheek" appearance.** It is characterized by an eruption that presents initially as an erythematous malar blush followed by an erythematous maculopapular eruption on the extensor surfaces of extremities that evolves into a reticulated, lacy, mottled appearance. Fever and other symptoms may be present but are uncommon. In patients with **chronic hemolytic anemias** like sickle-cell disease, **aplastic anemia** is a serious complication. Pregnant women should avoid exposure to this virus, since it may cause fetal hydrops in 10% of cases.

Sickle-cell patients can develop osteomyelitis (**a**), however, the clinical presentation is inconsistent. Patients with osteomyelitis caused by *Salmonella* species are generally those with sickle-cell disease. However, the most common organism that causes osteomyelitis in patients with sickle-cell disease is *S aureus*. Encephalitis (**b**) is an inflammation of the brain parenchyma and is not commonly caused by parvovirus. Common etiologic agents include herpes simplex, herpes zoster, varicella-zoster, West Nile virus, and toxoplasmosis. Pneumonia (**c**) is a common diagnosis in patients of all ages. In children, the most common causative agents are viral. The most commonly found bacterial agent is *S pneumonia*. Meningitis (**e**) is an infection of the meninges that surround the brain. It is caused by viral and bacterial entities. The most common bacterial agents include: *E coli*, group B *Streptococcus*, and *L monocytogenes* in very young infants and *S pneumonia*, *N meningitides*, and *H influenza* in older children.

4-33. The answer is b. (*Ropper, pp 39, 50.*) Groups of muscle fibers are innervated by individual motor neurons. Characteristically, these muscle fibers will exhibit similar properties on histochemical staining with ATPase, phosphorylase, oxidases, and other markers of cellular characteristics. Adjoining groups of muscle fibers in skeletal muscle may have very different histochemical staining characteristics, but they are usually similar in size. With denervation, all the muscle fibers supplied by the damaged neuron or axon will atrophy. These atrophied fibers may recover if they are reinnervated by branches from adjacent neurons that have not been damaged.

4-34. The answer is a. (*Brunicardi, pp 518-519.*) Squamous cell carcinoma of the lip is the most common malignant tumor of the lip and constitutes 15% of all malignancies of the oral cavity. Basal cell carcinomas do occur on the lip, but much less frequently. There is a strong association between squamous cell tumors of the lip and sun exposure. Therefore, these lesions are more common in the southern United States and in occupational groups who work outdoors. Because of its greater sun exposure, the lower lip is the site of more than 90% of such lesions. Persistent hyperkeratosis precedes 35% to 40% of these lesions. The incidence of metastases increases with the size of the lesion, and spread is usually via lymphatics to the ipsilateral submental node. Contralateral nodal metastases are rare unless the lesion crosses the midline. Approximately 10% to 15% of all patients have metastases at the time of diagnosis. These lip tumors are very responsive to radiotherapy, which works well for small- to medium-sized lesions. Large lesions treated with radiotherapy usually require surgical reconstruction. Radiotherapy should not be used in patients who will have ongoing sun exposure to the area because radiation therapy sensitizes the tissues to solar trauma.

4-35. The answer is e. (*Fauci, p 3.*) The concept being advanced here is medication error. A new emphasis is being placed on reducing all medical errors, including those related to misreading of handwriting, which might include avoidance of certain abbreviations or use of an electronic medical record. In this case the pharmacist and/or nurse mistook the medication orders for one tablet po qd (orally once a day) for one tablet po qid (orally four times a day), such that the patient had received three doses of each antihypertensive by 6 PM. Other abbreviations to avoid include qhs (write "at bedtime" instead), QOD (write "every other day"), U ("write "unit"), and MS (write "morphine sulfate"). There is no particular clue to the other listed answers. For example, an allergic reaction would seem unlikely with medications previously well tolerated; there are no symptoms or signs of acute pulmonary embolism, and a prophylactic anticoagulant is in use. Hypovolemia would be unlikely to develop after admission in a patient receiving IV fluids. Vasovagal reaction would be associated with bradycardia.

4-36 to 4-39. The answers are 36-c, 37-d, 38-a, 39-b. *(Hay, pp 840-844, 848, 874. Kliegman, pp 2004, 2020-2023, 2032-2037, 2090. McMillan, pp 1698, 1699-1703, 2442. Rudolph, pp 1531-1534, 1536-1540, 1561.)* Howell-Jolly bodies (slide C) are small, spherical, nuclear remnants seen in the reticulocytes and, rarely, erythrocytes of persons who have no spleen (because of congenital asplenia or splenectomy) or who have a poorly functioning spleen (eg, in hyposplenism associated with sickle-cell disease). Ultrafiltration of blood is a unique function of the spleen that cannot be assumed by other reticuloendothelial organs.

A target cell is an erythrocyte with a membrane that is too large for its hemoglobin content; a thin rim of hemoglobin at the cell's periphery and a small disk in the center give the cell a target-like appearance. Target cells, which are more resistant to osmotic fragility than are other erythrocytes, are seen in children who have α-thalassemia, hemoglobin C disease, or liver disease (eg, obstructive jaundice or cirrhosis). Thalassemia major (slide D) presents in the second 6 months of life with severe anemia requiring transfusion, heart failure, hepatosplenomegaly, and weakness. Later, the typical facial deformities (maxillary hyperplasia and malocclusion) can be seen in a patient inadequately transfused. The diagnosis can be made on peripheral blood smear by the presence of poorly hemoglobinized normoblasts in addition to target cells in the peripheral blood.

Uniformly small microspherocyte (less than 6 μm in diameter) are typical of hereditary spherocytosis (slide A). Because of a decreased surface to volume ratio, these osmotically fragile RBCs have an increased density of hemoglobin. Although spherical RBCs also can appear in other hemolytic states (eg, immune hemolytic anemia, microangiography, ABO incompatibility, and hypersplenism), their cellular volume is only irregularly augmented. Patients with hereditary spherocytosis can present in the newborn period with anemia, hyperbilirubinemia, and reticulocytosis. They may remain asymptomatic until adulthood, when they develop symptoms. After infancy, hepatosplenomegaly and gallstones are common.

Although hemoglobin C disease (slide B) is frequently a mild disorder, target cells constitute a far greater percentage of total RBCs than in thalassemia major. In the heterozygous state, no anemia or disease is noted, but target cells are seen. In the homozygous state, a moderately severe hemolytic anemia, reticulocytosis, and splenomegaly are seen, along with a smear containing a large number of target cells.

4-40 to 4-46. The answers are 40-e, 41-g, 42-n, 43-j, 44-a, 45-k, 46-m. *(Kaplan, pp 202-203.)* In distortion, the external reality is grossly rearranged to conform to internal needs. Repression is the expelling or withholding of an idea or feeling from consciousness. This defense differs from suppression by affecting conscious inhibition of impulses to the point of losing and not just postponing goals. Reaction formation refers to the substitution of an unacceptable feeling or thought with its opposite. Sublimation is the achieving of impulse gratification and the retention of goals by altering a socially objectionable aim or object to a socially acceptable one. Sublimation allows instincts to be channeled rather than blocked or diverted. Sublimation is a mature defense, together with humor, altruism, asceticism, anticipation, and suppression. Somatization is the conversion of psychic derivatives into bodily symptoms and reacting with somatic manifestations rather than psychic ones. Intellectualization is the excessive use of intellectual processes to avoid affective expression or experience. Isolation of affect is the splitting or separation of an idea from the affect that accompanies it but that is repressed. Introjection is the internalization of the qualities of an object. When used as a defense, it can obliterate the distinction between the subject and the object. Projection is the perception of and reaction to unacceptable inner impulses and their derivatives as though they were outside the self. Identification with the aggressor is the adoption of characteristics or behavior of the victim's aggressor as one's own. For example, it is not uncommon for the victim of child abuse to grow up to be an abusive parent him- or herself. Projective identification occurs mostly in borderline personality disorder and consists of three steps: (1) an aspect of the self is projected onto someone else, (2) the projector tries to coerce the other person to identify with what has been projected, and (3) the recipient of the projection and the projector feel a sense of oneness or union. Denial is the avoidance of awareness of some painful aspect of reality by negating sensory data. Displacement refers to the shifting of an emotion or a drive from one object to another (eg, the shifting of unacceptable aggressive feelings toward one's parents to the family cat).

Block 5

Answers

5-1. The answer is c. (*Fauci, pp 2375-2376.*) This patient has vitamin D deficiency, a common cause of secondary osteoporosis, as diagnosed by the suboptimal serum 25,OH vitamin D level. Vitamin D deficiency at less than 15 ng/mL can lead to low bone density. Vitamin D deficiency leads to impaired intestinal absorption of calcium and lower serum calcium levels. The low serum calcium causes elevated iPTH. In order to maintain serum calcium homeostasis, calcium is sacrificed from the skeleton leading to low bone density. With increasing bone turnover alkaline phosphatase levels can be increased. With significant vitamin D deficiency the following pattern is characteristic: elevated iPTH, normal ionized calcium, and elevated alkaline phosphatase. The patient with uncomplicated postmenopausal osteoporosis (ie, primary osteoporosis) has normal iPTH, ionized calcium, and alkaline phosphatase levels.

5-2. The answer is e. (*McPhee, pp 370-397.*) The British Hypertension Society developed recommendations to help practitioners devise an optimal treatment regimen when combining antihypertensives. They recommend that persons younger than 55 years who are not black start an ACE inhibitor as first-line therapy (A). β-Blockers (B) can be used in this group, but are no longer considered ideal first-line therapy. In persons older than 55 years or black, the first-line therapy is either a calcium channel blocker (C) or a diuretic (D). If one medication does not control the blood pressure, the next step is to add an agent from the other category. For example, if you have an "A" or "B" medication, add a "C" or "D" medication. If that still doesn't control the blood pressure, use A (or B) + C + D. Those still resistant should consider an α-blocker or other agent.

5-3. The answer is b. (*Brunicardi, p 1696.*) The radiograph demonstrates a transverse fracture of the distal half of the humeral shaft. The radial nerve runs in a groove on the posterior aspect of the humerus as it courses into the forearm compartment and is therefore at high risk of injury. If the nerve injury is apparent before any manipulation has been done, the fracture should be reduced; the nerve injury should be observed, since the nerve function will likely improve with time. If the nerve injury is present only after reduction, immediate surgical exploration is warranted because the nerve might be trapped in the fracture site. At this level of the arm, the ulnar and median nerves are well protected by muscle. The posterior interosseous nerve is a distal branch of the radial nerve and may be injured in fractures near the radial head, but it is in no danger from injuries at the level seen in this radiograph. There is no ascending circumflex brachial nerve.

5-4. The answer is d. *(Mahutte.)* The negative predictive value is the probability that a negative test correctly identifies an individual who does not have the disease. Using a 4 × 4 chart:

	Disease present	Disease absent	Total
Test positive	A = 10	B = 0	10
Test negative	C = 10	D = 80	90
Total	20	80	**100**
Negative predictive value = D/(C+D), or 80/90 = 89%			

5-5. The answer is a. *(Kaplan, pp 137-140.)* Although the relationships between emotional deprivation and failure to thrive are complex, the fact that children who are emotionally deprived do not grow well even when an adequate amount of food is available, is well proven. Renée Spitz studied institutionalized children and demonstrated that, due to lack of adequate nurturing, they become apathetic, withdrawn, and less interested in feeding, which in turn causes failure to thrive and, in extreme cases, death. Spitz called this syndrome anaclitic depression. Schizophrenia and autism have not been associated with emotional deprivation in infancy.

5-6. The answer is c. *(Fauci, pp 818-821.)* The diagnosis is very consistent with *C difficile* disease. The patient is elderly, has been in both a nursing home and hospital setting and received more than a week of a fluoroquinolone antibiotic. Mild fever, abdominal pain, and watery diarrhea are all consistent with the diagnosis, and the cell culture cytotoxicity test is the most specific of diagnostic tests. Failure on metronidazole is increasingly reported with at least a 25% failure rate. Switch to oral vancomycin is recommended. The patient does not have fulminant disease which usually presents as an acute abdomen, sepsis, or toxic megacolon. Synthetic fecal bacterial enema is one potential treatment being studied for recurrent *C difficile* disease but is not standard treatment.

5-7. The answer is d. *(Hay, pp 413-414, 1062-1067. Kliegman, pp 970-975. McMillan, pp 2423-2427. Rudolph, pp 1177-1179.)* Eczema is a chronic dermatitis that occurs in a population with a strong personal or family history of atopy. The skin presents initially as an erythematous, papulo-vesicular, weeping eruption, which progresses over time to a scaly, lichenified dermatitis. From about 3 months to about 2 years of age, the rash is prominent on the cheeks, wrists, scalp, postauricular areas, and arms and legs. In a young child 2 to 12 years of age, mainly the extensor surfaces of arms, legs, and neck are involved. Pruritus is a predominant feature, and scratching leads to excoriation, secondary infection, and lichenification of the skin. The rash has a chronic and relapsing course, and treatment is determined by the major clinical features. Cutaneous irritants (bathing in hot water, scrubbing vigorously with soap, wearing wool or synthetic clothing) should be avoided, and maximal skin hydration with emollients is essential. Topical moisturizers, steroids, and topical calcineurin inhibitors (tacrolimus and pimecrolimus) are the mainstays of therapy for atopic dermatitis. The use of antihistamines can provide additional relief from pruritus.

5-8. The answer is b. *(Mengel, pp 108-112.)* The history described is classic for primary dysmenorrhea. Oral contraceptive pills are an appropriate choice for treatment. They work by suppressing menstrual fluid volume and prostaglandin release, but not synthesis. This is achieved through endometrial hypoplasia. NSAIDs decrease prostaglandin production. Oral contraceptives do not increase vasoconstriction of the uterus or directly impact uterine tone.

5-9. The answer is a. *(Fauci, pp 1665-1668, 1684-1688.)* Bilevel positive airway pressure (BiPAP) ventilation has found increased favor in acute lung or heart disease, especially in those with acute CO_2 retention. The use of BiPAP may prevent the need for endotracheal intubation with its concomitant risks. BiPAP is contraindicated in patients with severe respiratory acidosis, decreased level of consciousness, bradypnea, or hemodynamic instability, for whom endotracheal intubation is the best treatment. Although oxygen should never be withheld from a hypoxic patient, caution must be exercised in patients with chronic CO_2 retention. Overly aggressive oxygen therapy may actually increase $PaCO_2$. In patients with chronic CO_2 retention, a targeted oxygen saturation of 88%-92% is appropriate. Admission to the ICU is appropriate, but the patient must be stabilized before transporting. Antibiotics are given for severe COPD exacerbations (especially if the patient is producing purulent sputum) but will not affect the immediate outcome of his respiratory failure.

5-10. The answer is c. *(Brunicardi, pp 46, 52-53.)* Bile and the fluids found in the duodenum, jejunum, and ileum all have an electrolyte content similar to that of Ringer lactate. Saliva, gastric juice, and right colon fluids have high K^+ and low Na^+ content. Pancreatic secretions are high in bicarbonate. It is important to consider these variations in electrolyte patterns when calculating replacement requirements following gastrointestinal losses.

5-11. The answer is a. *(Ropper, pp 606-609.)* There are many bases for abscess formation in the brain, but the most frequent causes are blood-borne infections from sources in the lung, heart, sinuses, and ears. Extension of infection from a chronic otitis or mastoiditis was much more common before the introduction of antibiotics. Facial or dental infections may spread to the brain through valveless veins draining about the muscles of mastication and communicating with the venous drainage of the brain.

5-12. The answer is e. *(Fauci, pp1417-1419.)* The patient in question has symptomatic tachycardia-bradycardia syndrome. Sinus node automaticity is suppressed by the tachyarrhythmia and results in a prolonged sinus pause following termination of the tachycardia. The patient in this case is symptomatic, and pacemaker placement is warranted; reassurance would put the patient at risk of further syncopal episodes and bodily harm from fall or accident. Although a pacemaker will prevent bradycardia, it does not prevent tachycardia. The patient may need medication to prevent tachycardia if she continues to be symptomatic after pacemaker placement. It is unlikely that any positive findings on a stress test could be correlated with her ECG findings. The tachy-brady syndrome does increase the patient's risk of cardioembolic event, and anticoagulation should be considered. Aspirin, however, is not an appropriate agent to prevent cardioembolic disease.

5-13. The answer is d. *(Mengel, pp 37-43.)* This case describes the classic distribution of scabies. Sarcoptes scabiei burrow into intertriginous areas, wrists, or areas where clothing is tight next to the skin. The lesions of chigger bites are similar, but bites are typically found in a linear pattern over wrists, ankles, and legs. Bedbugs typically infest unclothed areas—the neck, hands, and face. Fleas typically bite the lower extremities, and lesions from body lice would not follow the pattern described.

5-14. The answer is b. *(Jacobson, pp 116-117.)* Phencyclidine (PCP) intoxication is characterized by neurological, behavioral, cardiovascular, and autonomic manifestations. Intoxicated patients are often agitated, enraged, aggressive, and scared. Because of their exaggerated and distorted sensory input, they may have unpredictable and extreme reactions to environmental stimuli. Nystagmus and signs of neuronal hyperexcitability (from increased deep tendon reflexes to status epilepticus) and hypertension are typical findings.

5-15. The answer is d. *(O'Brien, 2007.)* The patient's presentation is consistent with **alcoholic ketoacidosis (AKA).** This is an acute metabolic acidosis that typically occurs in people who (1) chronically abuse alcohol and have a **recent history of binge drinking,** (2) have had little or **no recent food intake,** and (3) have had persistent vomiting. AKA is characterized by elevated serum ketone levels and a high anion gap ($\uparrow$AG = Na − [HCO3 + Cl] > 12). A concomitant metabolic alkalosis is common, secondary to vomiting and volume depletion. AKA is the result of (1) starvation with glycogen depletion and counterregulatory hormone production; (2) a raised NADH/NAD+ ratio (related to the metabolism of ethanol); and (3) volume depletion, resulting in ketogenesis. The typical symptoms and physical findings relate to volume depletion and chronic alcohol abuse and include nausea, vomiting, abdominal pain, and/or hematemesis. The fruity odor of ketones may be present on the patient's breath. The patient's mental status may be impaired. Also associated with the presentation are dyspnea, tremulousness, and dizziness. Rarely do patients present with muscle pain, fever, diarrhea, syncope, seizure, or melena. In AKA, the β-hydroxybutyrate (β-OH)/ acetyl acetate (AcAc) formation ratio is 5:1. The nitroprusside reaction (Acetest) may be negative or only weakly positive for serum ketones because nitroprusside reacts with AcAc, but not with β-OH. Therefore, ketosis may be more severe than would be inferred from a nitroprusside reaction alone.

Once the diagnosis of alcoholic ketoacidosis is established, the **mainstay of treatment is (b) hydration with 5% dextrose in normal saline (D$_5$NS or $^1/_2$; NS).** With initial therapy, ketone formation shifts toward the production of AcAc so that measured ketone levels rise, although β-OH levels decrease. Carbohydrate and fluid replacement reverse the pathophysiologic derangements that lead to AKA by increasing serum insulin levels and suppressing the release of glucagon and other counterregulatory hormones. Dextrose stimulates the oxidation of NADH and aids in normalizing the NADH/NAD+ ratio.

As additional treatment, thiamine supplementation should be given as prophylaxis against Wernicke encephalopathy. In general, exogenous insulin is contraindicated in the treatment of AKA because it may cause life-threatening hypoglycemia in patients with depleted glycogen stores.

Fluids alone (a, b, and c) do not correct AKA as quickly as fluids and carbohydrates combined, thus making the type of solution quite relevant (e) to managing this patient indeed.

5-16. The answer is b. (*Hay, p 1044. Kliegman, p 2221. McMillan, pp 405-406, 1850-1851. Rudolph, p 1639.*) Oligohydramnios can cause a number of serious problems in the infant, including constraint deformities (such as clubfoot) and pulmonary hypoplasia. These infants have usually experienced intrauterine growth retardation and frequently have an associated serious renal abnormality. Ultrasound of the kidneys is important to rule out renal involvement as a cause of the oligohydramnios. None of the other testing would be expected to identify an etiology for the oligohydramnios and pulmonary hypoplasia, although this child's ultimate clinical course might necessitate additional testing. The finding of bilateral renal agenesis is termed Potter sequence.

5-17. The answer is d. (*Fauci, pp 2301-2302.*) The classification of diabetes mellitus has changed to emphasize the process that leads to hyperglycemia. Type 2 DM is a group of heterogeneous disorders characterized by insulin resistance, impaired secretion of insulin, and increased glucose production. In this type 2 patient, the first intervention, medical nutrition therapy, failed to achieve the goal HgA1c of < 7.0%. *Medical nutrition therapy* (MNT) is a term now used to describe the best possible coordination of calorie intake, weight loss, and exercise. It emphasizes modification of risk factors for hypertension and hyperlipidemia, not just weight loss and calorie restriction. Blood glucose control should be evaluated after 4 to 6 weeks and additional therapy should be added; therefore, continued observation is not the best option. Metformin is considered first-line therapy in that it promotes mild weight loss, has known efficacy and side effect profile, and is available as a generic with very low cost. Thiazolidinediones ("glitazones"), sulfonylureas, and insulin are considered second line or add-on therapy for most patients with type 2 DM.

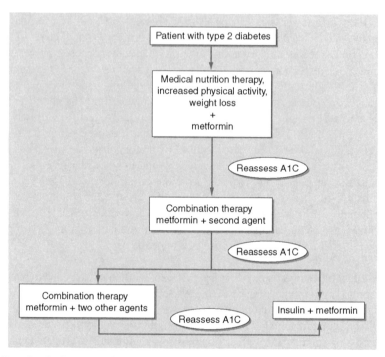

(Reproduced, with permission, from Fauci A et al. Harrison's Principles of Internal Medicine, 17th ed. New York, NY: McGraw-Hill, 2008.)

5-18. The answer is a. (*Cunningham, pp 498-500, 519-520. Beckmann, pp 105-107.*) The patient is having adequate uterine contractions as determined by the intrauterine pressure catheter. Therefore, augmentation with Pitocin is not indicated. The patient's diagnosis is secondary arrest of labor, which requires cesarean section. In the active phase of labor, a multiparous patient should undergo dilation of the cervix at a rate of at least 1.5 cm/h if uterine contractions are adequate. There is no indication for the use of vacuum or forceps in this patient because the patient's cervix is not completely dilated and the head is unengaged. Assisted vaginal delivery with vacuum or forceps is indicated when the patient is completely dilated, to augment maternal pushing when maternal expulsive efforts are insufficient to deliver the fetus. It is not recommended to continue to allow the patient to labor if dystocia is diagnosed, because uterine rupture is a potential complication.

5-19. The answer is c. (*Hay, pp 500-502. Kliegman, pp 1763-1766. McMillan, pp 694-695. Rudolph, pp 1275-1277.*) The description is that of croup. This infection involves the larynx and trachea; it usually is caused by parainfluenza or respiratory syncytial viruses. The usual age range for presentation is 6 months to 6 years. Symptoms include low-grade fever, barking cough, and hoarse, inspiratory stridor without wheezing. The pharynx can be normal or slightly red, and the lungs are usually clear. In children in severe respiratory distress, prolonged dyspnea can progress to physical exhaustion and fatal respiratory failure. Expiratory stridor is usually associated with a fixed obstruction, such as a tumor or vascular ring. Because agitation can be a sign of hypoxia, sedation should not be ordered. Hyperinflation on chest x-ray is seen in asthma, not croup. One condition in the differential in this child is epiglottitis, a now rare disease owing to widespread use of the *H influenza* b vaccine. Its presentation is more abrupt, with higher fever in rather toxic-appearing patients.

5-20. The answer is d. (*Mengel, pp 121-126.*) In 85% of women with recurrent UTIs, symptoms develop within 24 hours of sexual intercourse. If measures like voiding after intercourse, acidification of the urine, and discontinuing diaphragm do not work, prophylaxis is indicated for women with frequent infections. Single-dose postcoital antibiotic use is often helpful. If that does not decrease infections, daily single dose antibiotic prophylaxis may be appropriate for 3 to 6 months. If symptoms reoccur after discontinuation of daily prophylaxis, it may need to continue for 1 to 2 years.

5-21. The answer is c. (*Fauci, p 383, 1610*) The clues to this diagnosis are recurrent urinary tract infections and the use of suppressive therapy to control these infections. Nitrofurantoin is commonly used for this purpose. Nitrofurantoin can cause an acute hypersensitivity pneumonitis. This condition can progress to a chronic alveolitis with pulmonary fibrosis. The presenting symptoms are fever, chills, cough, and bronchospasm. In addition, the patient may experience arthralgias, myalgias, and an erythematous rash. The chest x-ray will show interstitial or alveolar infiltrates. CBC often shows leukocytosis with a high percentage of eosinophils. The treatment is to discontinue the nitrofurantoin, and begin corticosteroids. Sepsis secondary to a urinary tract infection, and a healthcare-related pneumonia might be considered. However, these would not present with a diffuse erythroderma or eosinophilia. Acute bacterial infections cause a neutrophilic leukocytosis; eosinophils are usually undetectable owing to the stress effect of catecholamines and cortisol. COPD rarely presents in a 30 year old.

Lymphocytic interstitial pneumonia is a rare disease. Lung biopsy to establish the diagnosis of an interstitial lung disease would be considered only after the potentially offending drug had been discontinued.

5-22. The answer is d. (*Moore, pp 590-595.*) There are multiple findings on chest x-ray that are suggestive of a thoracic aortic injury, such as widening of the mediastinum more than 8 cm (because of the presence of a mediastinal hematoma), loss of the aortic knob, deviation of the nasogastric tube in the esophagus, depression of the left mainstem bronchus, an apical cap (apical pleural hematoma), sternal or scapular fracture, multiple left-sided rib fractures, and massive left hemothorax. However, a normal chest x-ray does not rule out a diagnosis of a thoracic great vessel injury. If clinical suspicion is high, then further diagnostic workup should be pursued. Aortography, CT angiography, and transesophageal echocardiography may establish the diagnosis. Traumatic aortic injuries are deceleration injuries because of differential forces to the fixed and mobile parts of the thoracic aorta; most aortic injuries are located near the ligamentum arteriosus.

5-23. The answer is d. (*Ropper, pp 1037, 1130, 1132.*) The "Mad Hatter" of *Alice in Wonderland* was a familiar site in the nineteenth century. Persons who cured felt (used in the manufacture of hats) with nitrate of mercury often developed pronounced personality changes, tremor, and ataxia. This type of poisoning is now more typically seen in paper, pulp, and electrochemical plants that use phenyl mercury as part of the manufacturing process. Pathologic changes in the CNS are usually prominent in the cerebellum and include extensive damage to the granular cell layer of the cerebellum. The calcarine cortex of the occipital lobe is also especially vulnerable, and damage to this tissue correlates with constriction of the visual fields.

5-24. The answer is a. (*Ropper, pp 1034-1036.*) Decorative paint and glazes manufactured and sold outside the United States may have very high lead levels. Even mildly acidic solutions, such as orange juice, may leach enough lead out of the paint to produce symptoms in persons exposed over a protracted period to fluids contaminated with the lead. Bilateral neuropathies may develop in adults exposed to lead, and the radial nerves are the most common sites of damage. This neuropathy at its most severe form will produce wrist and finger drops as well as occasionally very mild sensory abnormalities in the distribution of the radial nerves. Signs associated with the lead neuropathy may include abdominal pain, constipation, anemia, basophilic stippling of erythrocyte precursors, and a linear discoloration along the gingival margin (lead lines). Penicillamine is used as a chelating agent to reduce the body load of lead.

5-25. The answer is b. (*Ropper, p 1036.*) Acute poisoning with arsenic may cause tonic-clonic seizures or a less dramatic encephalopathy. Hemolysis may be substantial and mucosal irritation may be evident. Death may develop with circulatory collapse if the dose of arsenic is substantial enough. The polyneuropathy that develops with chronic poisoning is resistant to treatment with chelating agents such as BAL. If the patient survives the poisoning, peripheral nerve damage resolves over the course of months or years.

5-26. The answer is f. (*Ropper, pp 1032-1033.*) This man's history suggests a nutritional disorder rather than poisoning, but his clinical picture is consistent with chronic ergotism. Ergot is a potent vasoconstricting agent derived from the rye fungus, *Claviceps purpurea*. Currently, the contamination of bread with this material is unlikely in developed nations, but it is still a problem in areas with antiquated agricultural techniques. Chronic ergot poisoning is associated with histologic changes in the CNS, which include degeneration of the posterior columns and dorsal roots. A peripheral neuropathy is also evident, but persons at risk for this disorder are also at risk for other nutritional disturbances that may produce neuropathy.

5-27. The answer is c. (*Ropper, p 1036.*) Manganese inhalation by miners produces a clinical picture similar to that seen with hepatolenticular degeneration (Wilson disease). Parkinsonism is the most prominent feature, but axial rigidity and dystonia may also develop. Neuronal loss is evident in several areas of the brain, including the globus pallidus, putamen, caudate, hypothalamus, and cerebellum. Treatment with L-dopa is usually less effective with this heavy metal injury than it is with Parkinson disease. Agents more likely to produce parkinsonism in the general population include phenothiazines, butyrophenones, and metoclopramide. Metoclopramide (Reglan) is used increasingly after gastrointestinal surgery to manage nausea and other signs of gastrointestinal irritability. Although most physicians do ask about exposure to reserpine-like medications or phenothiazines, other drugs that may cause parkinsonism in susceptible persons are sometimes overlooked.

5-28. The answer is e. (*Ropper, pp 963-964.*) Carbon monoxide (CO) poisoning can be seen in victims of fires, in those who attempt suicide by carbon monoxide inhalation, or in those who are otherwise exposed to the gas in an unventilated setting. Because of its greater affinity for hemoglobin than oxygen, CO reduces oxygen in the blood and leads to prolonged hypoxia and acidosis. Symptoms may range from confusion and headache at carboxyhemoglobin levels of 20% to coma, posturing, and seizures at levels of 50% to 60%. Characteristic of CO poisoning is delayed neurologic deterioration occurring 1 to 3 weeks after the initial event. Typically, this takes the form of an extrapyramidal disorder with parkinsonian gait and bradykinesia. Imaging may show the classic hypodensities in the globus pallidum bilaterally.

5-29. The answer is a. *(Rosen, pp 1293-1295.)* The test is the **Obturator sign,** in which the patient is supine with the right thigh flexed; passive internal or external rotation of the hip eliciting pain is a positive test for **appendicitis.** The pain is attributed to an inflamed appendix that is irritated by stretching the obturator internus muscle.

(**b**) The psoas sign for appendicitis is tested by having the patient lie on his or her left side; pain caused by passive right hip extension is a positive result. (**c**) Rovsing sign refers to pain in the RLQ elicited by palpation in the LLQ. (**d**) McBurney point is the classic location of maximum tenderness to palpation in the RLQ, one-third the distance from the anterior superior iliac crest to the umbilicus. It is common in patients with an anterior appendix. (**e**) Murphy sign refers to pain causing cessation of respiration during palpation of the RUQ and is seen in acute cholecystitis.

5-30. The answer is c. *(Mengel, pp 273-277.)* The test described in this question is called the straight leg raising test. The test is considered positive when the patient feels pain below the knee when the leg is raised 30° to 60°. The positive test indicates nerve root irritation, likely because of a herniated disk. A back strain should not produce a positive straight leg raising test. A compression fracture may occur suddenly, but would be unlikely in an otherwise healthy young man. Neoplasms and inflammatory conditions would be less likely to occur suddenly.

5-31. The answer is d. *(Katz, pp 148-152. ACOG Guidelines for Women's Health Care, pp 145-158.)* It would be appropriate for this patient to receive a hepatitis B vaccination, since it is recommended for all individuals with a history of multiple sexual partners. She is not a candidate for the varicella vaccine since she has had chicken pox. The hepatitis A vaccine is indicated for international travelers, illegal drug users, and health care workers. The pneumococcal vaccine is indicated in immunocompromised persons, those with chronic illnesses, and individuals more than 65 years old. The influenza vaccine is especially indicated in pregnant women, individuals with chronic diseases, and those in long-term-care facilities.

5-32. The answer is b. (*Fauci, pp 2083-92, 2149-58.*) Despite the negative rheumatoid factor, this patient has rheumatoid arthritis. Rheumatoid factors, which are autoantibodies reactive with the Fc portion of IgG, are present in more than 2/3 of adults with the disease, but are not specific for rheumatoid arthritis. Anti-CCP is found in most patients with RA, and has a higher specificity than the measurement of rheumatoid factor. Vague musculoskeletal complaints are common early manifestations of RA. Early diagnosis and treatment are key to slowing the irreversible bony destruction caused by synovial inflammation. While physical therapy maintains joint strength and mobility, it will not mitigate the disease. Disease modifying antirheumatic drugs (DMARDs) are appropriate for early use, but their use requires experienced and well-educated practitioners. Therefore, the most appropriate next step in this patient who has failed nonsteroidal anti-inflammatory drugs is referral to a rheumatologist for DMARD initiation. There is no indication for allopurinol without the diagnosis of gout, or for doxycycline without the diagnosis of Lyme disease.

5-33. The answer is a. (*Hay, pp 1276-1280. Kliegman, pp 313-316. McMillan, pp 63-66. Rudolph, pp 1644-1646, 1650-1652.*) Initial bolus therapy in the emergency center should have been with isotonic fluid such as normal saline or lactated Ringer solution. Slow correction of this hypernatremia (more than 24-48 hours) prevents significant fluid shifts and increased intracranial pressure. Hyperglycemia may be seen in hypernatremic dehydration because of decreased insulin secretion and cell sensitivity to insulin; this is particularly important to recognize because increased serum glucose can cause the serum sodium to be falsely decreased. Blood products such as fresh-frozen plasma are not indicated, and rapid infusion of hypotonic solutions such as D10W and $^1/_4$; normal saline could cause rapid fluid shifts resulting in cerebral edema and death. Hypertonic (3%) saline is used only in the event of seizures caused by rapid rehydration (or in children with hyponatremic dehydration and associated central nervous system symptoms), along with other emergent measures typically used to reduce cerebral edema.

5-34. The answer is b. (*Hay, pp 32-34. Kliegman, p 681. McMillan, pp 200-201. Rudolph, pp 82, 99, 105, 168, 207.*) There is loss of body weight of 1.5% to 2% per day for the first 5 days of life for a normal newborn infant as excessive fluid is excreted. One might think this would tend to cause hemoconcentration and produce an increase in hematocrit, but, to the contrary, the hematocrit falls as an adaptation to an environment of higher oxygen. Infants usually have several meconium stools during the first day or two of life, changing to soft yellow stools after 1 to 2 days of life. As the hematocrit falls, there is a corresponding increase in serum bilirubin that peaks around 3 to 5 days of life. Temperature should not change; temperature instability in a term infant is frequently a sign of serious infection.

5-35. The answer is b. (*Schwesinger, pp 411-416.*) *Helicobacter pylori* infections have become extremely common: nearly one-third of all American adults are now infected. Morphologically, the organism is a gram-negative, corkscrew-shaped, motile bacillus with three to seven flagella. Noninvasive approaches with simple, relatively inexpensive serologic and urea breath tests can establish the diagnosis of *H pylori* infection. Culturing endoscopic scrapings or biopsy specimens has proved to be impractical because of the need for special media and elaborate growth conditions. A rapid urease test is used when endoscopy provides a specimen for analysis. Therapy is problematic because the organism is not easily eradicated. Monotherapy is largely ineffective. Eradication of *H pylori* requires triple therapy with colloidal bismuth (Pepto-Bismol), an antibiotic (amoxicillin or ampicillin), and a nitroimi-dazole such as metronidazole. However, dual- and triple-drug therapy can achieve eradication in 80% to 90% of patients. Unfortunately, compliance rates with multidrug therapy are low.

5-36. The answer is c. (*Greenfield, pp 1187-1206.*) An indirect inguinal hernia leaves the abdominal cavity by entering the dilated internal inguinal ring and passing along the anteromedial aspect of the spermatic cord. The internal inguinal ring is an opening in the transversalis fascia for the passage of the spermatic cord; an indirect inguinal hernia, therefore, lies within the fibers of the cremaster muscle. A femoral hernia passes directly beneath the inguinal ligament at a point medial to the femoral vessels, and a direct inguinal hernia passes through a weakness in the floor of the inguinal canal medial to the inferior epigastric artery. Neither lies within the cremaster muscle fibers. Spigelian hernias, which are rare, protrude through an anatomic defect that can occur along the lateral border of the rectus muscle at its junction with the linea semilunaris. An interparietal hernia is one in which the hernia sac, instead of protruding in the usual fashion, makes its way between the fascial layers of the abdominal wall. These unusual hernias may be preperitoneal (between the peritoneum and transversalis fascia), interstitial (between muscle layers), or superficial (between the external oblique aponeurosis and the skin).

5-37. The answer is b. (*Kaplan, pp 1062-1062.*) The lithium level considered effective for acute mania is between 1 and 1.5 meq/L. Levels above 1.5 meq/L carry a risk of toxicity that outweighs the potential benefits. Lithium levels need to be interpreted in the context of the clinical presentation, because some patients, especially the medically ill and the elderly, may present with clear symptoms of lithium toxicity at levels below 1.5 meq/L.

5-38 to 5-40. The answers are 38-d, 39-b, 40-e. (*Fauci, pp 1752-1761.*) Acute renal failure in adults usually occurs during hospitalization for other illness. The history (in particular, exposure to nephrotoxins including intravenous contrast agents), physical examination (in particular, assessment of volume status and search for allergic manifestations such as skin rash), and urine studies will usually establish the diagnosis. The fractional excretion of sodium may demonstrate renal underperfusion if this is not clear from the clinical setting. If the kidneys are underperfused from volume depletion, third space losses or poor cardiac output, the kidneys will retain salt and water, and the fractional excretion of sodium (FENa) will be low. In the cases presented here, the clinical setting suggests the diagnosis.

Interstitial nephritis typically occurs as an allergic reaction to antibiotics, particularly beta-lactams and sulfa derivatives. So-called tubular proteinuria is modest (<1 g/24 h), albuminuria is minimal and the nephrotic syndrome does not occur. Pyuria and eosinophiluria are usually present. The commonest cause of acute renal failure is acute tubular necrosis. The FENa is usually above two and muddy brown cases may be present on the urinalysis. Ischemia (often owing to sepsis) and nephrotoxins are the usual causes. Obstructive uropathy can occur acutely, particularly in the setting of bladder outlet obstruction (BPH) or neurogenic bladder (as can occur in diabetes). The patient will often have difficulty voiding and the urinalysis will be unremarkable. Complete anuria or fluctuations from oliguria to polyuria also suggest the diagnosis. Bladder catheterization or renal sonography are diagnostic.

5-41. The answer is e. (*Tintinalli, pp 198-199.*) **WPW syndrome** is caused by an **accessory electrical pathway (ie, Bundle of Kent)** between the atria and ventricles. The primary significance of WPW syndrome is that it predisposes the individual to the development of reentry tachycardias. The classic ECG findings include a **short PR interval (< 120 msec)**, **widened QRS interval (> 100 msec)**, and a **delta wave** (slurred upstroke at the beginning of the QRS). When conduction occurs anterograde down the AV node and then retrograde up the accessory pathway (orthodromic), the ECG will appear normal. When the impulse occurs anterograde down the accessory pathway and retrograde up the AV node (antidromic), the QRS complex will be wide. In the presence of antidromic conduction (conduction first through the bypass tract), the normal slowing effect of the AV node is lost and rapid ventricular response rates (> 200 beats per minute) can occur. The most dangerous circumstance is in atrial fibrillation where impulses occur at a rate greater than 300 beats per minute. This can quickly lead to ventricular fibrillation.

(a) Ventricular tachycardia may be difficult to distinguish from WPW. In a young patient with classic ECG findings, however, WPW is more likely. Nonetheless, it is prudent to avoid AV nodal blocking agents in any wide complex tachycardia. (b) Atrial flutter will have flutter waves that take on a sawtooth pattern. (c) Atrial fibrillation is an irregular rhythm. (d) LGL syndrome is classified as a preexcitation syndrome (similar to WPW) in which a bypass tract is present. LGL is characterized by an individual who is prone to tachydysrhythmias and has a PR interval less than 120 msec. Unlike WPW, the QRS complex is normal (no delta wave).

5-42. The answer is c. (*Beckmann, pp 289-292.*) The degree or severity of pelvic relaxation is rated on a scale of 1 to 3, based on the descent of the organ or structure involved. First-degree prolapse involves descent limited to the upper two-thirds of the vagina. Second-degree prolapse is present when the structure is at the vaginal introitus. In cases of third-degree prolapse, the structure is outside the vagina. Total procidentia of the uterus is the same as a third-degree prolapse, which means that the uterus would be located outside the body.

5-43. The answer is d. (*Jacobson, pp 154-156.*) Hypochondriasis is recognized by the patient's preoccupation with having a serious medical condition based on the misinterpretation of his or her own bodily symptoms. Despite medical evaluation and reassurance, the patient continues to fear that the disease is present. Often, after reassurance is given (usually because a negative test result is received) the patient is temporarily relieved, but this relief does not last. The symptoms must cause clinically significant distress, and be present for longer than 6 months.

5-44. The answer is c. (*Jacobson, pp 154-156.*) The patient should be referred to a primary care doctor who will see her regularly but not perform any invasive procedures unless there is a clear indication to do so. New complaints or fears about an illness should be dealt with by the primary care physician, using a limited evaluation (history or physical examination) to ensure that no organic disease has developed, since even patients with hypochondriasis can become physically ill. Since these patients do not believe that their disorder is psychiatric, referral for psychotherapy is likely to be unsuccessful. The patient in this question reports no other signs of depression, and thus an antidepressant is not warranted. Likewise, though she has a recurrent complaint/concern about ovarian cancer, this does not rise to delusional proportions—she is capable of being reassured, at least for a time, by negative results. Presuming the patient has already had a work-up for ovarian cancer, which it appears by history that she has, further work-up for this disease is unwarranted.

5-45. The answer is c. (*Rosen, pp 2119-2124.*) The crystallized free base of cocaine is known as "crack cocaine." This form, smoked through a pipe, produces a highly lipid-soluble vapor that allows for rapid transport from the lungs to the brain for a quicker high compared to cocaine that is snorted or injected. As a result of this mechanism, the substance can be concentrated in high amounts in the lung parenchyma causing an **infiltrative inflammatory process** and **pneumonitis** referred to as "crack lung." This can subsequently result in respiratory failure.

Cannabis (**a**) used in conjunction with inhaled β_2-agonists may result in bleb formation and subsequent pneumothorax, but not pneumonitis. Opioids (**b**), methamphetamine (**d**), and alcohol (**e**) may have pulmonary effects through secondary mechanisms, but are not primarily responsible for this type of presentation.

5-46. The answer is d. (*Ropper, pp 24-25.*) The artery of Adamkiewicz is a major anterior radicular artery and may supply the lower two-thirds of the spinal cord. It is at risk of occlusion during abdominal aortic aneurysm repair. Other branches of the aorta or internal iliac arteries may also supply the thoracic and lumbar cord. The upper segments of the spinal cord are usually supplied off the vertebral arteries.

Block 6

Answers

6-1. The answer is b. (*American Academy of Family Physicians, 2008.*) In general, colorectal cancer screening should begin at age 50. In cases where there is a family history of colorectal cancer, the screen should begin 10 years before the cancer was diagnosed in the family, or at age 50, whichever is sooner.

6-2. The answer is a. (*Ropper, pp 939-940.*) Electromyogram and nerve conduction studies are a way to establish anterior horn cell damage. The conduction times would be normal even with extensive motor neuron disease, but the pattern of spontaneous and evoked muscle potentials would be abnormal.

6-3. The answer is c. (*Hay, pp 967-968. Kliegman, pp 2260-2261. McMillan, pp 1831-1832. Rudolph, pp 1740-1742.*) The child in the photograph has an undescended testis, or cryptorchidism. By 6 months of life, 0.8% of boys born at term still have cryptorchidism. In adults with cryptorchidism, the risk of testicular malignancy is much higher than in unaffected men. Orchiopexy does not eliminate this risk, but repositioning the testes makes them accessible for periodic examinations. Whether the testes are brought into the scrotum or not, the sperm count can be reduced. The failure of the testes to develop, and their subsequent atrophy, can be detected by 6 months of age. Torsion of the testis is a potential risk because of the excessive mobility of the undescended testis. Orchiopexy helps to eliminate this problem. The incidence of UTI and epididymitis are not affected by the position of the testes.

6-4. The answer is e. (*Brunicardi, pp 1508-1510.*) Wilms tumor is the most common abdominal malignancy of childhood, but represents only about 10% of childhood malignant tumors. This is a nephroblastoma (Wilms tumor) adherent to the left kidney. These tumors are associated with aniridia (rarely) and with hemihypertrophy, cryptorchidism, or hypospadias in about 10% of cases. Most patients present with an asymptomatic mass found by a parent. Less than one-third of patients experience hematuria. As would be expected in over half such cases, this child is hypertensive, probably due to compression of the renal artery by the mass. Surgical treatment consists of resection of the kidney and ureter. Chemotherapy is indicated in patients with malignancy confined to one kidney, and chemoradiation is indicated after surgical excision for more advanced disease. Cure rates exceeding 80% are achieved in patients with hematogenous metastases. CT scan is used to assess the tumor characteristics and evaluate for metastases. Ultrasonography is utilized to assess for vascular invasion into the renal vein or vena cava.

6-5. The answer is b. (*Rosen, pp 388-391, 1000-1005.*) **Inspiratory and expiratory radiographs** allow better visualization of the lung pleura and may help better elucidate the presence of a pneumothorax not initially visualized on the chest radiograph.

A repeat chest x-ray **(a)** may be performed; however it will be low-yield if the original was performed correctly. A chest CT scan **(c)** may be done, but after the proper films are performed. Chest thoracostomy **(d)** involves placing a tube inside the pleural cavity to evacuate the intrapleural air and may be performed if the patient continues to decompensate and if the suspicion for a pneumothorax remains high. Chest thoracotomy **(e)** involves opening the chest cavity and is reserved for the severest cases of cardiovascular collapse.

6-6. The answer is d. (*Moore and Jefferson, pp 265-266.*) Neuroleptic malignant syndrome (NMS) is a relatively rare but potentially fatal complication of neuroleptic treatment. Its main features are hyperthermia, severe muscular rigidity, autonomic instability, and changes in mental status. Associated findings are increased CPK, increased liver transaminase activity, leukocytes, and myoglobinuria. The mortality rate can be as high as 30% and can be higher when the syndrome is precipitated by depot forms. Neuroleptic malignant syndrome is more common in young males when high-potency neuroleptics are used in high doses and when dosage is escalated rapidly. The first step in management of NMS is discontinuation of all antipsychotic medications. Supportive treatments include treatment of extrapyramidal symptoms with antiparkinson medications, correcting fluid imbalances, treating fever, and managing hypertension or hypotension. Dopaminergic agents such as dantrolene, bromocriptine, and amantidine are used in the treatment of more severe cases.

6-7. The answer is a. (*Fauci, pp 1485-1486, 2430-2431.*) The patient's history of sickle cell disease should raise the suspicion of iatrogenic iron overload. Multiple transfusions in a patient whose anemia is not attributed to blood loss lead to tissue iron accumulation and end organ damage just like genetic hemochromatosis. Measures to assess body iron status (transferrin saturation, serum ferritin level) are the initial diagnostic studies. This patient's diabetic status may also be related to iron accumulation. Evidence of cardiomegaly (from physical examination and chest x-ray) together with a low voltage on ECG suggests an infiltrative process affecting the heart. Brain-natriuretic peptide (BNP) is released from the cardiac myocytes in response to ventricular stretch and can be a useful tool in determining whether someone is suffering from heart failure. BNP will not, however, help determine the cause of the heart failure. Holter monitoring and cardiac catheterization are not necessary in patients without evidence of intermittent arrhythmias or coronary ischemia respectively. CT of the chest is used to assess lung nodules or parenchymal abnormalities (such as interstitial lung disease) but would not be useful in this patient with clear lung fields on CXR.

6-8. The answer is a. (*Ropper, pp 1068-1070.*) Spinal cord ischemia is usually most severe in the distribution of the anterior spinal artery. The posterior spinal artery is more a plexus of arteries with extensive anastomoses than a discrete pair of blood vessels running along the dorsal aspect of the spinal cord. With a lesion of the spinal cord from ischemia or pressure, the spinothalamic tracts, which are responsible for pain and temperature perception and for providing information for two-point discrimination and graphesthesia, are more vulnerable to injury than are the posterior columns. The posterior columns, which are primarily responsible for vibration and position sense, are supplied by the posterior spinal arteries.

6-9 to 6-10. The answers are 9-d, 10-a. (*Jacobson, pp 153, 157, 159.*) Factitious disorder usually presents with physical or mental symptoms that are induced by the patient to meet the psychological need to be taken care of (primary gain). These patients will often mutilate themselves repeatedly in a frantic effort to be cared for by the hospital system. Moving between hospitals so that they don't get caught is common, especially when the patient is directly confronted. Malingering is similar to factitious disorder in that symptoms are faked, but the motive for malingering is some secondary gain, such as getting out of jail. Somatization disorder is characterized by the recurrent physical complaints that are not explained by physical factors and that cause significant impairment or result in seeking medical attention. Pain of any part of the body and dysfunctions of multiple systems are typical. The *DSM-IV* diagnostic criteria for somatization disorder include at least four pain symptoms, one sexual symptom, and one pseudoneurological symptom. These symptoms can be present at any time in the duration of the disorder. Somatization disorder usually emerges in adolescence or the early twenties and follows a chronic course. Somatization disorder is diagnosed predominantly in women, with a prevalence of 0.2% to 0.5%, and rarely in men. Body dysmorphic disorder is characterized by distorted beliefs about the patient's own appearance, often with delusional qualities. Borderline personality disorder patients may mutilate themselves, but the object is generally to get attention or relieve stress.

6-11. The answer is e. (Meisel, 2006.) In general, young people presenting with chest pain do not increase suspicion for myocardial ischemia, but when historical features are appropriate, it must be considered. While a family history of heart disease is a risk factor for myocardial ischemia, it is less likely in this very young patient. "Heartburn" is not a feature suggestive of myocardial ischemia. A recent viral infection may precede an episode of pericarditis or myocarditis, either of which could present with severe chest pain, but this does not increase suspicion for ischemia. His smoking history is certainly significant, but not as important as his history of drug use given his age. His physical examination findings (diaphoresis and agitation) are more consistent with a stimulant use, likely cocaine. The risk of myocardial infarction increases 24 times that of baseline in the 60 minutes after cocaine use.

6-12. The answer is e. (Ropper, pp 1058-1059.) Rabies is usually spread through the saliva of an infected animal. Introduction of saliva into a bite wound allows the virus to inoculate muscles or subcutaneous tissues. After introduction of the virus, the incubation period until fulminant infection appears extends from a few days to over 1 year, but usually ranges from 1 to 2 months. Bites of the head and face carry the greatest risk of causing fatal disease. Early after exposure, the patient will often complain of pain or paresthesias at the site of the animal bite. Animals transmitting the virus include dogs, bats, skunks, foxes, and raccoons. Dehydration as a complication of rabies is no longer likely because intravenous fluids can be given to completely replace what the hydrophobic patient cannot consume by mouth. Other complications of rabies include a paralytic form of the disease that progresses to quadriplegia (dumb rabies) in 20% of patients. With the classic form of the disease, the patient will also exhibit intermittent hyperactivity.

6-13. The answer is e. (Hay, pp 836-837. Kliegman, pp 2006-2009. McMillan, pp 1707-1709. Rudolph, pp 1566-1567.) This child has transient erythroblastopenia of childhood (TEC), the most common acquired RBC aplasia in children. This condition is commonly diagnosed between the ages of 1 to 3 years and some affected children have a history of a recent viral infection;

however, no specific virus has been implicated (parvovirus B19 is usually specifically excluded). Physical findings are minimal and include pallor and tachycardia. Laboratory studies reveal a profound anemia and reticulocytopenia with a marked reduction in erythrocyte precursors in the marrow. RBC adenosine deaminase (ADA) levels are normal. The condition lasts for several months, and may require 1 or 2 transfusions, but ultimately is self-limited. Steroids are not helpful.

Alternative diagnoses with this presentation include Diamond-Blackfan anemia (DBA), but this condition is congenital and usually presents in infancy; RBC ADA levels are usually elevated. In addition, about half of patients with DBA will have congenital anomalies including short stature, cranial abnormalities, and upper extremity abnormalities. Pearson marrow-pancreas is another form of congenital hypoplastic anemia, including poor growth, pancreatic fibrosis with insulin-dependant diabetes, and muscle and nerve involvement. Early death is typical. Sickle-cell patients usually have evidence of ongoing hemolysis on their smear, and iron deficiency causes a microscopic hypochromic anemia.

6-14. The answer is c. (*Tintinalli, p 356.*) **Sildenafil (Viagra)** is a selective cyclic guanosine monophosphate (GMP) inhibitor that results in smooth-muscle relaxation and vasodilation by the release of nitric oxide. It is used in men for erectile dysfunction. It is **contraindicated to administer nitroglycerin** to individuals who have taken sildenafil in the previous 24 hours. The combination of nitroglycerin and sildenafil can lead to hypotension and death. If nitrates are coadministered with sildenafil, the patient should be closely monitored for hypotension. Fluid resuscitation and pressor agents may be needed to restore BP.

(**a**) Aspirin is contraindicated in individuals with an anaphylactic allergy or active bleed. (**b**) Heparin is contraindicated in individuals with heparin-induced thrombocytopenia, and those who are actively bleeding. (**d**) Metoprolol is contraindicated in hypotensive individuals. (**e**) Morphine sulfate is contraindicated in patients with respiratory depression.

6-15. The answer is c. (*Rakel, pp 1339-1345.*) Opiate withdrawal is well-characterized, and although not life-threatening in otherwise healthy adults, can cause severe discomfort. Symptoms from a short-acting drug like heroin can occur within just a few hours. Withdrawal from longer acting opiates may not cause symptoms for days. Early symptoms include lacrimation, rhinorrhea, yawning, and diaphoresis. Restlessness and irritability occur later, with bone pain, nausea, diarrhea, abdominal cramping, and mood lability occurring even later.

Cocaine does not have a significant physiologic withdrawal syndrome, but craving is intense. Marijuana-withdrawal syndrome is also not physiologically significant. Ecstasy can be considered a hallucinogen or a stimulant, and withdrawal is often associated with depression, but not the symptoms described above. Benzodiazepine withdrawal mimics alcohol withdrawal, and is associated with hypertension, tachycardia, and possibly seizures.

6-16. The answer is d. (*Cunningham, pp 373-387, 537, 539, 889-890.*) Post-term or prolonged pregnancies are those pregnancies that have gone beyond 42 completed weeks of gestation. In general, obstetricians do not allow pregnancies to persist after 42 weeks because of the significantly increased incidence of perinatal morbidity and mortality. If a patient has a ripe cervix, it is reasonable to induce the patient at 41 weeks because the chance of having a successful vaginal delivery is very high. On the other hand, if the patient has an unripe cervix, it is generally recommended that she continue with the pregnancy. Alternatively, a patient can be induced at 41 weeks with an unripe cervix if cervical ripening agents are used. If a patient waits until 42 weeks and still has an unripe cervix, then admission with administration of cervical ripening agents prior to Pitocin induction is recommended to improve the likelihood of a successful vaginal delivery. The Bishop score is a way to determine the favorability of the cervix to induction. The elements of the Bishop score include effacement, dilation, station, consistency, and position of the cervix (see table). Points are assigned for each element, and then totaled to give the Bishop score. Induction to active labor is usually successful with a Bishop score of 9 or greater. In the scenario described here, the patient has a Bishop score of 4, which is unfavorable for induction. Therefore, expectant management is a reasonable management plan to try to give the cervix time to ripen to avoid a cesarean section. It is not recommended to perform an elective section without a trial of labor because of the risks of major surgery.

BISHOP SCORE					
Points	Dilation	Effacement	Station	Consistency	Position
0	Closed	0%-30%	−3	Firm	Posterior
1	1-2 cm	40%-50%	−2	Medium	Midposition
2	3-4 cm	60%-70%	−1, 0	Soft	Anterior
3	≥ 5 cm	≥ 80%	+1, +2	—	—

6-17. The answer is d. (*Townsend, pp 1603-1606.*) The patient most likely has an infected pancreatic pseudocyst. Pseudocysts are nonepithelialized fluid collections that can present at earliest 4 to 6 weeks after an episode of acute pancreatitis. The treatment for infected pancreatic pseudocysts is similar to that for pancreatic abscesses—percutaneous catheter drainage with antibiotics. Aspiration of the fluid can be diagnostic but is not a definitive treatment, even with the addition of antibiotics. Internal drainage of pancreatic pseudocysts is contraindicated in the presence of infection but is the treatment of choice for mature, symptomatic, noninfected pseudocysts. Malignancy should be excluded if there is no preceding history of pancreatitis.

6-18 to 6-20. The answers are 18-d, 19-c, 20-a. (*Fauci, pp 2233-2238.*) In a young female with hyperthyroidism, low or absent radioiodine uptake in the thyroid and a coexisting pelvic mass, you should consider struma ovarii (ectopic thyroid tissue in a teratoma of the ovary). Whole body radionuclide scanning can demonstrate ectopic thyroid tissue. Surreptitious use of thyroid supplements (factitious hyperthyroidism) can occur in healthcare workers who have access to thyroid hormone. Classic symptoms of hyperthyroidism occur and the serum T_4 is elevated. Radioactive iodine uptake would show subnormal values, as there is no thyroid hormone production in the gland itself. The thyroid gland is not palpable. A tender thyroid gland and elevated ESR make subacute thyroiditis a likely diagnosis. Hyperthyroid symptoms are common early in the illness. The condition is self-limited (usually lasting 6-8 weeks); so antithyroid drugs are not used. Beta-blockers can alleviate symptoms until the inflammation resolves.

6-21. The answer is b. (*Brunicardi, p 52.*) This patient's history of tinnitus in conjunction with her mixed metabolic acidosis-respiratory alkalosis is pathognomonic of salicylate intoxication. Salicylates directly stimulate the respiratory center and produce respiratory alkalosis. By building up an accumulation of organic acids, salicylates also produce a concomitant metabolic acidosis. The patient is in a state of metabolic acidosis as shown by a markedly increased anion gap of 28 mEq unmeasured anions per liter of plasma. However, the respiratory response is greater than can be explained by a compensatory response; respiratory compensation alone would not result in an alkalemic pH. The disturbance cannot be pure respiratory alkalosis, since the serum bicarbonate does not drop below 15 mEq/L as a result of renal compensation and the anion gap does not vary by more than 1 to 2 mEq/L from its normal value of 12 in response to a respiratory disturbance. The renal response to hyper-ventilation involves wasting of bicarbonate and compensatory retention of chloride; it does not involve a change in the concentration of unmeasured anions, such as albumin and organic acids.

Phenformin and methanol overdoses also produce high-anion-gap metabolic acidosis, but without the simultaneous respiratory disturbance. Sedatives, such as barbiturates or diazepam, would result in hypoventilation with respiratory acidosis.

6-22. The answer is a. (*McPhee, pp 1150-1177.*) Prophylaxis against *M avium* complex (MAC) should be instituted once the patient's CD4 count drops below 75 to 100 lymphocytes/mm^3. Prophylaxis against *Pneumocystis* pneumonia should be considered once the CD4 count drops below 200 lymphocytes/mm^3. Prophylaxis for fungal disease has been studied, but there was no benefit in the group that had prophylaxis with regard to mortality. Prophylaxis for herpes simplex and herpes zoster is not generally done. CMV prophylaxis can be instituted in those with CMV IgG positivity and with CD4 counts below 50 lymphocytes/mm^3, but it is generally not done because ganciclovir (the primary prophylactic agent) can cause neutropenia.

6-23. The answer is d. (*Kaplan, pp 390-407.*) A diagnosis of alcohol dependence requires the presence of compulsive drinking with ineffective attempts to stop or cut down (the housewife in this vignette has tried to "limit her alcohol intake but without success"); evidence of a severe impairment of occupational, social, and family life because of the great amount of time the patient spends procuring and consuming alcohol or recovering from its effects (she has not been able to take part in several important family events because she was too ill or did not want to miss her nightly drinking); persistent excessive drinking despite the problems alcohol causes (she has continued to drink despite these issues); and physical symptoms and signs of withdrawal and tolerance (shakiness and anxiety when she misses a drink).

6-24. The answer is a. (*Swaiman, p 82.*) On shining a light through the pupil of the normal newborn, the normal color of the retina is perceived as an orange-red reflection of the light. Failure to perceive that reflection usually indicates opacification of the pathway of light transmission. Several types of intrauterine infections, including rubella and CMV infection, may produce congenital cataracts and impair light transmission in this way. The presence of a distinctive white reflex usually indicates disease behind the lens, such as a scar from retinopathy of prematurity or a retinoblastoma.

6-25. The answer is c. *(Hay, p 960. Kliegman, p 2348. McMillan, p 2078. Rudolph, pp 2154-2155.)* Hypercalcemia can develop in children who are immobilized following the fracture of a weight-bearing bone. Serious complications of immobilization hypercalcemia, and the hypercalciuria that occurs as a result, include nephropathy, nephrocalcinosis, hypertensive encephalopathy, and convulsions. The early symptoms of hypercalcemia—namely, constipation, anorexia, occasional vomiting, polyuria, and lethargy—are nonspecific and may be ascribed to the effects of the injury and hospitalization. Therefore, careful monitoring of these patients with serial measurements of the serum ionized calcium and the urinary calcium to creatinine ratio is critical during their immobilization. A ratio of greater than 0.2 establishes a diagnosis of hypercalciuria. Although complete mobilization is curative, additional measures, such as vigorous intravenous hydration with a balanced salt solution, dietary restrictions of dairy products, and administration of diuretics, can be instituted. For patients who are at risk for symptomatic hypercalcemia, short-term therapy with calcitonin is highly effective in reducing the concentration of serum calcium by inhibiting bone resorption.

6-26. The answer is a. *(McPhee, pp 121-123.)* Treatment for warts should be geared toward inducing "wart-free" intervals for as long as possible, and trying not to create scarring. No treatment can guarantee a remission or absolutely prevent reoccurrences. All the therapies listed in this question may be used for warts, but topical liquid nitrogen is the best choice in this case. Podophyllum resin should not be used during pregnancy. Imiquimod is often used for anogenital warts, but has not demonstrated benefit for common warts. Laser therapy is effective, but leaves open wounds that heal by secondary intention and should be reserved for warts resistant to other treatment modalities. Bleomycin injection has a high cure rate, but shouldn't be used on digital warts because of potential complications including terminal digital necrosis.

6-27. The answer is d. *(Rosen, pp 1272-1276.)* The patient's clinical picture is consistent with **acute pancreatitis.** Ranson developed criteria that help **predict mortality rates** in patients with pancreatitis. The presence of more than three criteria equals 1% mortality, while the presence of six or more criteria approaches 100% mortality. **Ranson criteria** at admission are age > 55, WBC > 16,000, glucose > 200, LDH > 350, AST > 250. Within 48 hours of admission, hematocrit fall > 10%, BUN rise > 5, serum calcium < 8, arterial PO_2 < 60, base deficit > 4, and fluid sequestration > 6 L. The patient in the case fulfills four of Ranson criteria and has approximately

15% mortality risk. Note that lipase and amylase are not part of Ranson criteria despite being relevant in the diagnosis of acute pancreatitis.

6-28. The answer is b. *(Fauci, pp 158-162.)* Delirium is a common complication in the hospital setting. Delirium may be differentiated from dementia by its acute onset and waxing and waning mental state. Elderly patients, especially those with a history of dementia, and the severely ill are at greatest risk of developing delirium. Delirium may be precipitated by medications, postsurgical state, infection, or electrolyte imbalance. The management of delirium relies on nonpharmacologic approaches, including frequent reorientation, discontinuation of any unnecessary noxious stimuli (eg, urinary catheters, unnecessary oxygen delivery systems or telemetry monitors, and restraints), environmental modification to establish day/night sleep cycles, and discontinuation of all unnecessary medications. This patient likely will continue to need pain control, but the dose of fentanyl should be minimized to the smallest effective dose. Benzodiazepines frequently induce a delirium and their continued use or escalation may impair recovery. Fluoroquinolones can worsen mental status in the elderly. Physical or chemical restraints actually impair recovery from delirium and should be used only as last resort to prevent serious harm to self or others. A repeat urinalysis would provide no useful information since the original urine culture is still pending.

6-29. The answer is d. *(Hay, pp 521-523, 1197-1200. Kliegman, pp 1240-1254. McMillan, pp 1142-1155. Rudolph, pp 949-959.)* The key to controlling tuberculosis in children and eradicating the disease is early detection and appropriate treatment of adult cases; the child, once infected, is at lifelong risk for the development of the disease and for infecting others, unless given appropriate prophylaxis. The usual source of the disease is an infected adult, since smaller children are not infectious because they typically are unable to produce enough intrathoracic pressure with a cough to spread the disease. Household contacts of a person with newly diagnosed active disease have a considerable risk of developing active tuberculosis, and the risk is greatest for infants and children. Therefore, when tuberculosis is diagnosed in a child, the immediate family and close contacts should be tested with tuberculin skin tests and chest radiographs and treated appropriately when indicated. Bronchoscopy would be indicated only in unusual circumstances. Three to eight weeks is required after exposure before hypersensitivity to tuberculin develops. This means that the tuberculin test must be repeated in exposed persons if there is a negative reaction at the time that contact with the source of infection is broken. TB skin tests are usually negative in infants of this age, even when active disease is ongoing. A logical preventive measure is the administration of isoniazid to the 6-week-old baby for 3 months when a Mantoux (purified protein derivative, PPD) can then be placed. Transmission of tuberculosis occurs when bacilli-laden, small-sized droplets are dispersed into the air by the cough or sneeze of an infected adult. Small children with primary pulmonary tuberculosis are not considered infectious to others, and they are not capable of coughing up and producing sputum. Sputum, when produced in child of this age, is promptly swallowed, and for this reason specimens for microbial confirmation can be obtained by means of gastric lavage from smaller children.

In the child described in the case, the chest film is abnormal, suggesting active TB disease. While the medications listed in the answer are part of the treatment for TB disease, they are typically used with several other medications.

6-30. The answer is d. (*Ropper, pp 915-925.*) The tremor is of a parkinsonian type. The patient also has the classic findings of Parkinson disease: asymmetric tremor, rigidity, and bradykinesia. Parkinson disease is primarily the result of loss of dopaminergic cells in the substantia nigra and other pigmented nuclei. Cerebral cortex is commonly involved in epilepsy which is characterized by repeated unprovoked seizures. Guillain-Barré syndrome is a peripheral demyelinating disease that usually presents as an ascending motor deficit. Multiple sclerosis is a central nervous system (CNS) demyelinating disease, involving cerebral white matter. It presents with individual episodes of CNS deficits, which usually recover to some extent. Cerebellar dysfunction may cause a tremor, but not rigidity and bradykinesia.

6-31. The answer is a. (*Kaplan, p 912.*) The first order of business with a physically violent patient is to ensure the safety of the patient and the caregivers. Since this patient has already been physically violent, it is not the time to reason with the patient verbally, or offer medication orally. The patient should be put immediately in full leather restraints (not soft restraints). Since medical students and residents are rarely fully trained in the safe restraint of a violent patient, this is better done by those that are trained if at all possible.

6-32. The answer is b. (*Brunicardi, pp 31-32.*) The misconception that the entire bowel does not function in the early postoperative period is still widely held. Intestinal motility and absorption studies have clarified the patterns by which bowel activity resumes. The stomach remains uncoordinated in its muscular activity and does not empty efficiently for about 24 hours after abdominal procedures. The small bowel functions normally within hours of surgery and is able to accept nutrients promptly, either by naso-duodenal or percutaneous jejunal feeding catheters or, after 24 hours, by gastric emptying. The colon is stimulated in large measure by the gastro-colic reflex but ordinarily is relatively inactive for 3 to 4 days. Well-nourished patients who undergo uncomplicated surgical procedures can tolerate up to 10 days without full nutritional support before significant problems with protein breakdown begin to occur. Enteral nutrition is preferred over par-enteral nutrition because of decreased risks of nosocomial infections and catheter-related complications.

6-33. The answer is e. *(Fauci, pp 1983-1990.)* Cirrhosis caused by hepatitis C is the most common cause for liver transplantation in the United States. A previous history of alcoholism is not a contraindication to transplantation, although most transplant centers require abstinence from alcohol for 6 months before transplantation is considered. Three-year survival rate after transplan-tation in most centers now exceeds 80%. The model for end-stage liver dis-ease (MELD) scoring system is used in the United States to allocate cadaveric livers to potential donors. Patients with complications of cirrhosis (esophageal variceal bleeding, hepatic encephalopathy, and uncontrolled ascites) or who have significantly elevated bilirubin, INR, and serum creati-nine are usually made eligible for transplantation. Repeat liver biopsy would be unnecessary and potentially risky due to the patient's coagulopathy. Patients with end-stage cirrhosis from hepatitis C do not benefit from inter-feron and ribavirin therapy.

6-34. The answer is e. *(Moore and Jefferson, p 198.)* Derealization is the sub-jective sense that the environment is strange or unreal, as if reality had been changed. Perception is a physical sensation given a meaning or the integra-tion of sensory stimuli to form an image or impression; in dulled perception, this capacity is diminished. Retardation of thought refers to the slowing of thought processes that may be seen in major depression. Response time to questions may be increased. Depersonalization refers to feeling that one is falling apart or not one's self, that one's self is unreal or detached.

6-35. The answer is b. *(Selwyn, 2005.)* The patient's clinical presentation is consistent with **Prinzmetal or variant angina.** This condition is caused by focal **coronary artery vasospasm.** It **occurs at rest** and exhibits a **circadian pattern,** with most episodes occurring in the early hours of the morning. The pain commonly is severe. Distinguishing unstable angina related to coronary atherosclerosis from variant angina may be difficult and requires special investigations, including coronary angiography. Patients may also exhibit ST elevations on their ECGs. Nitrates and CCBs are the mainstays of medical therapy for variant angina. Nitroglycerin effectively treats episodes of angina and myocardial ischemia within minutes of administration, and the long-acting nitrate preparations reduce the frequency of recurrent events. CCBs effectively prevent coronary vasospasm and variant angina, and they should be administered in lieu of β-blockers. **(a)** Aspirin is an antiplatelet agent that helps reduce progression of plaque formation in the coronary arteries. Aspirin won't treat the vasospasm that is responsible for variant angina. **(c)** β-Blockers can be beneficial in patients with fixed coronary artery stenosis and exertional angina. However, for variant angina, nonselective β-blockers may be detrimental in some patients because blockade of the β-receptors, which mediate vasodilation, allows unopposed β-receptor–mediated coronary vasoconstriction to occur, thus possibly causing an actual worsening of symptoms **(d)** H_2-blockers are used to treat acid reflux symptoms. **(e)** The etiology of the patient's symptoms will not be relieved by an antidepressant.

6-36. The answer is d. (*South-Paul, pp 289-297.*) The mainstay of therapy for cluster headaches is to provide relief from the acute attacks, then use therapy to suppress headaches during the symptomatic period. Nifedipine has been shown to be effective, as has prednisone, indomethacin, and lithium. However, the medication should not be given daily, just during the symptomatic period. Fluoxetine has not been shown to be beneficial, and ergotamine is generally only helpful in the acute stage—not for prophylaxis.

6-37. The answer is d. (*Greenfield, pp 1728-1729.*) The patient's presentation of acute onset, persistent back pain, and hypotension is classic for ruptured abdominal aortic aneurysm. The CT scan reveals a fractured ring of calcification in the abdominal aorta with significant density (blood) in the para-aortic area. The incidence of ischemic colitis following abdominal aortic repair is about 2%. The incidence dramatically increases following a ruptured aneurysm repair. The sigmoid colon is affected most frequently. Blood flow to the left colon is normally derived from the IMA with collateral flow from the middle and inferior hemorrhoidal vessels. The SMA may also contribute via the marginal artery of Drummond. If the SMA is stenotic or occluded, flow to the left colon will be primarily dependent on an intact IMA. The IMA is usually ligated at the time of aneurysm repair. Patients at highest risk for diminished flow through collateral vessels are those with a history of visceral angina, those found to have a patent IMA at the time of operation, those who have suffered an episode of hypotension following rupture of an aneurysm, those in whom preoperative angiograms reveal occlusion of the SMA, and those in whom Doppler flow signals along the mesenteric border cease following occlusion of the IMA. Bowel ischemia recognized at the time of operation should be treated by reimplantation of the IMA into the graft to restore flow.

6-38. The answer is b. *(Hay, pp 529-530. Kliegman, p 2180. McMillan, p 1439. Rudolph, p 1998.)* The patient in the question has a classic description of Goodpasture syndrome, a rare disease in children. The pulmonary hemorrhage can be life threatening and the renal function progressive. Diagnosis is suggested by kidney biopsy and finding antibodies to the glomerular basement membrane.

Hemolytic-uremic syndrome presents in a child with fever, bloody diarrhea, and progression toward renal failure but not respiratory symptoms. Nephrotic syndrome presents with edema, hypertension, and proteinuria; respiratory symptoms related to congestive heart failure (and not pulmonary hemorrhage) might be seen. Poststreptococcal glomerulonephritis can result in hematuria, but the respiratory symptoms associated with the condition would be related to congestive heart failure and not to pulmonary hemorrhage. Renal vein thrombosis might result in hematuria but would not be expected to have pulmonary findings.

6-39 to 6-43. The answers are 39-e, 40-b, 41-d, 42-c, 43-a. *(Katz, pp 359-363.)* Bleeding occurs in about 30% to 40% of human gestations before 20 weeks of pregnancy, with about half of these pregnancies ending in spontaneous abortion. A threatened abortion takes place when this uterine bleeding occurs without any cervical dilation or effacement. In a patient bleeding during the first half of pregnancy, the diagnosis of inevitable abortion is strengthened if the bleeding is profuse and associated with uterine cramping pains. If cervical dilation has occurred, with or without rupture of membranes, the abortion is inevitable. If only a portion of the products of conception has been expelled and the cervix remains dilated, a diagnosis of incomplete abortion is made. However, if all fetal and placental tissue has been expelled, the cervix is closed, bleeding from the canal is minimal or decreasing, and uterine cramps have ceased, a diagnosis of complete abortion can be made. The diagnosis of missed abortion is suspected when the uterus fails to continue to enlarge with or without uterine bleeding or spotting. A missed abortion is one in which fetal death occurs before 20 weeks gestation without expulsion of any fetal or maternal tissue for at least 8 weeks thereafter. When a fetus is retained in the uterus beyond 5 weeks after fetal death, consumptive coagulability with hypofibrogenemia may occur. This is uncommon, however, in gestations of less than 14 weeks in duration.

6-44. The answer is d. (*Hay, p 1265. Kliegman, pp 856-857, 2262. McMillan, pp 1832-1833. Rudolph, pp 260-270.*) The patient in the question may have a torsion of his testis that requires immediate attention. Another possibility would be epididymitis, especially if there is a possible antecedent history of sexual activity or urinary tract infection. Prehn sign, although not totally reliable, is elicited by gently lifting the scrotum toward the symphysis. Relief of the pain points to epididymitis; its worsening, to torsion. Doppler ultrasound (or surgical consultation) is a logical first step in this man's evaluation, demonstrating absence of flow in torsion and increased flow in epididymitis. Alternatively, a radionuclide scan will show diminished uptake in torsion and increased uptake in epididymitis.

Treatment for torsion is surgical exploration and detorsion and scrotal orchiopexy. Causative organisms for epididymitis include *Neisseria gonorrhoeae, C trachomatis,* and other bacteria. Treatment with appropriate antibiotics and rest is indicated. However, treating this patient with antibiotics without first excluding testicular torsion is ill-advised; loss of the testis can be expected after 4 to 6 hours of absent blood flow if the testis has torsioned. Strangulated hernia is associated with evidence of intestinal obstruction.

6-45. The answer is a. (*Fauci, pp 1425, 1431.*) The rhythm strip reveals atrial flutter with 2:1 atrioventricular (AV) block. Management of atrial fibrillation or atrial flutter with rapid ventricular response is determined by the patient's hemodynamic stability. A hemodynamically unstable patient may require emergent cardioversion. In the stable patient, consideration should be given to initially controlling the ventricular response rate. This patient has a normal blood pressure and would probably respond to AV nodal blockade with metoprolol. Adenosine is also a nodal blockade agent, but its extremely short half-life limits its utility to diagnostic maneuvers. Amiodarone can be used to maintain NSR after cardioversion, but immediate management should focus on rate control. Chest compressions are inappropriate given the normal blood pressure.

6-46. The answer is b. (*Fauci, pp 668-671.*) The patient has probably had myelodysplastic syndrome (MDS) for years. This commonly causes anemia with mild macrocytosis in the elderly. Some of these patients will transform into acute myeloid leukemia. The leukemic cells can expand the marrow and cause diffuse bone pain (especially over the sternum and around the knees). Although 20% of patients with MDS may have mild splenomegaly, the newly detected spleen tip and the rapidly worsening pancytopenia suggest that leukemic cells are squeezing out the normal hematopoietic cells. Patients with secondary AML (ie, AML that arises from a preexisting hematopoietic disease) have a grave prognosis and respond poorly to combination chemotherapy. Folic acid deficiency would not cause leukocytosis. Viral infection and tuberculosis may present subacutely but not this chronically.

Block 7

Answers

7-1. The answer is d. *(Jacobson, pp 295-302.)* Autistic disorder is characterized by lack of interest in social interactions, severely impaired verbal and nonverbal communication, stereotyped behaviors, and a very restricted range of interests. Children with autism do not involve themselves in imaginative and imitative play and can spend hours lining and spinning things or dismantling toys and putting them together. Patients with obsessive-compulsive disorder may spend hours on repetitive tasks (such as lining up toys) but do not show the difficulties with language and social interaction that this patient displays. Patients with Asperger syndrome show no clinically significant delay in spoken or receptive language development, making this diagnosis unlikely. Patients with childhood disintegrative disorder have approximately a 2-year period of normal development (including speech and interpersonal skills) before this regresses; this patient has never apparently had such a period. Patients with Rett disorder by the age of 5 would be expected to have microcephaly and a disordered gait (unsteady and stiff).

7-2. The answer is b. *(Mengel, pp 121-126.)* Dysuria without pyuria is common. In the postmenopausal years, atrophy is a usual cause. In younger women, a careful history can reveal a bladder irritant (caffeine and acidic foods are common irritants). When hematuria is present, interstitial cystitis should be suspected. Interstitial cystitis is generally diagnosed through cystoscopy, based on the presence of ulcerations and fissures in the bladder mucosa and the absence of bladder tumors. Urodynamic studies often demonstrate a small bladder capacity, with urge to void with as little as 150 mL of fluid in the bladder.

7-3. The answer is b. *(Ropper, pp 915-925.)* Parkinson disease symptoms are due in large part to dopamine depletion. Carbidopa-levodopa can replete dopamine and alleviate symptoms. Alteplase is used to dissolve blood clots during acute strokes or heart attacks. Glatiramer and interferon β-1A are used to treat multiple sclerosis, and have been shown to decrease attacks. Both are thought to work through immunomodulation. Sertraline is a selective serotonin reuptake inhibitor. By increasing serotonin concentrations, it is effective for the treatment of depression.

7-4. The answer is c. (*Fauci, pp 115-117, 2572-2576.*) Cervical spondylosis (arthritis) or midline disc protrusion can cause cervical myelopathy, which can mimic amyotrophic lateral sclerosis. The neck pain and stiffness can be mild, and the patient can have both lower motor neuron signs such as atrophy, reflex loss, and even fasciculations in the arms and upper motor neuron signs such as hyperreflexia and clonus (from cord compression) in the legs. Therefore, the diagnosis of ALS is never made without imaging studies of the cervical cord, as compressive cervical myelopathy is a remediable condition. Disease in the cortex would never cause this combination of bilateral upper and lower neuron disease, so an MRI scan of the brain would be superfluous. Myopathies such as polymyositis or metabolic myopathy cause more proximal than distal weakness and would not be associated with hyperreflexia. You should think of disease of the neuromuscular junction (eg, myasthenia gravis) or muscle when the neurological examination is normal except for weakness. Simply referring the patient for physical or occupational therapy would leave her potentially treatable cervical spine disease undiagnosed. Decompressive surgery can improve symptoms and halt progressive loss of function in cervical myelopathy.

7-5. The answer is a. (*Fauci, pp 301, 322, 345.*) This patient's diffuse hair loss after a severe illness is caused by telogen effluvium. Normal hair follicles go through a life cycle. Approximately 5% are in the death (telogen) phase where the hair shaft is released. In telogen effluvium, the hair follicles are "shocked" by the systemic stress, and many enter the telogen phase at the same time. The diagnosis is made by careful history and physical examination. CBC, ANA, and hormonal levels will be normal. The patient will recover fully in a month or two, although a wig may be necessary to hide cosmetically troubling alopecia in the meantime. Diffuse hair loss may be seen with many drugs or with systemic illnesses such as hypothyroidism, systemic lupus, syphilis, or iron deficiency, but there is no evidence of any of these illnesses in this patient. Male pattern baldness (androgen-dependent alopecia) is seen in normal men, in some older women, and in women with androgen excess, but the hair loss affects the crown and frontal region rather than the scalp diffusely. The dramatic and acute hair loss of telogen effluvium does not occur in male pattern baldness.

7-6. The answer is d. (*Kaplan, p 821.*) Tumors of the pituitary cause bitemporal hemianopsia by compressing the optic chiasm and a variety of endocrine disturbances that in turn can cause psychiatric symptoms. woman in the question has a basophilic adenoma, and her depression part of her Cushing syndrome. Patients with craniopharyngiomas can als present with behavioral and autonomic disturbances caused by the upward extension of the tumor into the diencephalon.

7-7. The answer is c. *(Townsend, pp 692-693.)* Hemodialysis, rather than management by dietary manipulation alone, should be considered for patients with Stage 5 kidney disease defined as an estimated glomerular filtration rate of less than 15 mL/min/1.73 m² or earlier in patients with complications due to renal failure according to National Kidney Foundation guidelines. These complications include hyperkalemia, congestive heart failure, peripheral neuropathy, severe hypertension, pericarditis, bleeding, and severe anemia. The uremic hyperkalemic patient in congestive heart failure may require emergency dialysis in addition to the standard conservative measures, which include (1) limitation of protein intake to less than 60 g/day and restriction of fluid intake and (2) reduction of elevated serum potassium levels by insulin-glucose or sodium polystyrene sulfonate (Kayexalate) enema treatment. Arteriovenous fistulas require several weeks to months to develop adequate size and flow. While awaiting maturation, temporary dialysis can be satisfactorily performed using a catheter placed in a central vein. Renal biopsy would be performed in an attempt to obtain a diagnosis of the underlying renal disease. Patients who are acceptable candidates for kidney transplantation usually should undergo this form of treatment, after they are stabilized, rather than chronic hemodialysis, the mortality for which is now higher than for transplantation. Despite adequate dialysis, problems of neuropathy, bone disease, anemia, and hypertension remain difficult to manage. Compared with chronic dialysis, transplantation restores more patients to happier and more productive lives.

7-8. The answer is a. *(Ropper, pp 155-157.)* Oxygen may terminate a cluster headache within minutes. Some physicians recommend inhaling 4 L/min of 100% oxygen by mask as soon as signs of an impending headache develop. This has prompted many sufferers of cluster headaches to keep a cylinder of compressed oxygen at home during the season when they are most likely to develop such headaches. Cluster headaches usually occur at night when the patient is asleep, and so practical access to the oxygen tank is possible. Methysergide is effective in preventing cluster headaches for many persons, but it does rarely cause the worrisome adverse effect of fibrosis. Retroperitoneal, pulmonary, and endocardial fibroses are potential adverse effects of methysergide. Sublingual nitroglycerin may in fact trigger a headache and is not recommended for patients

..r headaches. Propranolol is a β-adrenergic–blocking ..n the prophylaxis of some vascular headaches, but it is ..orting a cluster headache. Dihydroergotamine supposito- ..t some vascular headaches, but they do not have as obvious ..cluster as in classic or common migraine syndromes.

The answer is b. (*Rosen, pp 120-122.*) The patient has a **progressive** .scending **peripheral neuropathy,** also known as **Guillain-Barré syndrome.** Patients can usually remember a preceding viral illness, usually gastroenteritis. **Deep tendon reflexes are typically absent.**

Hypokalemic periodic paralysis is part of the heterogeneous group of muscle diseases known as periodic paralyses and is characterized by episodes of flaccid muscle weakness occurring at irregular intervals. Most of the conditions are hereditary and are more episodic than periodic. Peripheral vascular disease **(c),** a common complication of longstanding diabetes, causes paresthesias in the distal lower extremities and not acute paralysis. Tetanus **(d)** manifests as muscular rigidity caused by the *Clostridium tetani* toxin preventing release of inhibitory neurotransmitters. Lockjaw is a common complaint in generalized tetanus. A brain abscess **(e)** typically presents with fever, headache, and focal neurologic findings and is usually caused by an associated trauma, surgery, or infectious spread from another site.

7-10. The answer is c. (*Rosen, pp 120-122.*) Progressive paralysis in Guillain-Barré syndrome can rapidly ascend to the respiratory system and cause **respiratory failure.** Patients need to be monitored and provided ventilator support as necessary.

(a) Guillain-Barré syndrome is a transient, not permanent, condition. **(b, d, and e)** are not complications of the syndrome.

7-11. The answer is b. (*Hay, pp 1262-1264. Kliegman, pp 857-858, 861. McMillan, p 587. Rudolph, pp 268-269.*) Pelvic inflammatory disease (PID) refers to sexually transmitted infections of the female upper genital tract including tubo-ovarian abscess, endometritis, salpingitis, and pelvic peritonitis. Each year, a diagnosis of PID is made in more than 1 million women. Sexually active teenagers are at great risk of acquiring PID because of their high-risk behavior, exposure to multiple partners, and failure to use contraceptives. The strong likelihood of PID in the patient presented should not preclude consideration of serious conditions requiring surgical intervention, such as appendiceal abscess, ectopic pregnancy, and ovarian cyst. Renal cyst does not present in the manner described. An episode of PID raises the risk of ectopic pregnancy, and about 20% of women become infertile following one episode of PID. Other sequelae include dyspareunia, pyosalpinx, tubo-ovarian abscess, and pelvic adhesions. Endometriosis is not related to PID.

7-12. The answer is e. *(Kaplan, p 1373.)* All states legally require that psychiatrists, upon becoming aware of a child who is the victim of sexual or physical abuse, report it to the appropriate state agency. In this case, some of the abuses occurred decades ago, and as such the victims are now probably adults. These cases would not require reporting to authorities. However, the active molestation of the 10-year-old boy requires reporting, since the harm to vulnerable children is considered to outweigh the rights of confidentiality in a psychiatric setting.

7-13. The answer is d. *(Fauci, pp 57-58.)* Falls in the elderly are common. Nearly one-third of community dwelling adults over 65 years of age fall at least once yearly. Minor imbalances are common in everyday life. Falling in the elderly is usually associated with decreased ability of the elderly to compensate for these imbalances. Age-related declines in vestibular function, autonomic function, hearing and eyesight, and muscular strength all contribute to the inability of the elderly to correct for minor imbalances. Medical illnesses and medications may also contribute to this difficulty. The evaluation of falling in the elderly includes a careful history to exclude syncope, a careful medication history, and a review of medical conditions, which may aggravate falling. Persons who have fallen more than once in the last 6 months are at high risk of falling again. The timed up-and-go (TUG) test also predicts who is likely to fall again in the next year. In an elderly person who presents with falling, evidence-based literature supports three measures to prevent future falls: elimination of medications with sedating and anticholinergic properties, elimination of environmental and structural hazards in the home, and physical therapy. Diphenhydramine has both sedating and anticholinergic effects.

In the absence of syncope and focal neurologic findings, CNS imaging, EEG and Holter monitoring are unnecessary. Since the patient does not have orthostatic hypotension, discontinuing HCTZ is not indicated. Donepezil is indicated for dementia but not just forgetfulness.

7-14. The answer is d. *(Townsend, p 2110.)* The CT findings are consistent with any of the suggested lesions. However, the most likely diagnosis in an immunocompetent patient is metastatic disease, which has an incidence of approximately 150,000 to 250,000 cases per year as compared to primary intracranial tumors, which have an incidence of 35,000 per year. Roughly 15% to 30% of cancer patients develop intracranial metastases during the course of their disease. The cancers that most frequently metastasize to the brain parenchyma include those of the lung, breast, kidney, gastrointestinal (GI) tract, and melanomas. Leukemia shows a predilection for the leptomeninges. A large majority of these lesions become symptomatic owing to mass effect from white matter edema. Treatment is dependent on the number and size of the lesions and the physical condition of the patient, but may include a combination of surgery, radiosurgery, and whole-brain radiation therapy. Immunocompromised patients are at increased risk for toxoplasmosis and central nervous system lymphomas. Both immunocompetent and immunocompromised hosts can develop pyogenic brain abscesses, which typically occur in the setting of known infection (which can spread either locally or hematogenously).

7-15. The answer is c. *(South-Paul, pp 533-542.)* In the case of an autosomal recessive trait, if unaffected parents have an affected child, there is a 25% risk that each offspring from those parents will be affected. Both parents must be carriers of the trait, which means that each child born to them has a 25% risk of not carrying the gene, a 50% risk of being a carrier, and a 25% risk of having the disease.

7-16. The answer is b. *(Hay, pp 612-613, 629-630. Kliegman, pp 1565-1567. McMillan, pp 373-375, 1920-1923. Rudolph, pp 1368-1370, 1461-1463.)* The radiograph demonstrates a stool-filled megacolon. Finding a dilated, stool-filled anal canal with poor tone on the physical examination of a well-grown child supports the diagnosis of functional constipation. Hirschsprung disease is usually suspected in the chronically constipated child despite 98% of such children having functional constipation. The difficulty in treating functional constipation, once it has been established as the diagnosis, emphasizes the need for prompt identification and treatment of problems with defecation and for counseling of parents regarding proper toileting behavior. An extensive workup of this patient would likely be negative and expensive, and is not indicated. Hirschsprung usually presents in infancy with increasingly difficult defecation in the first few weeks of life. Typically no stool is found in the rectum, and anal sphincter tone is abnormal. Diagnosis of Hirschsprung disease may be made with rectal manometry and rectal biopsy.

7-17. The answer is c. *(Ropper, pp 560-562.)* Kaposi sarcoma is unusually common in patients with AIDS, but it is rarely metastatic to the brain. Metastatic lymphomas producing meningeal lymphomatosis are not especially rare in the general population, but primary lymphomas (ie, lymphomas apparently arising in the CNS) were rare before the AIDS epidemic. The primary brain lymphoma usually presents as a solitary mass and can occur anywhere in the brain, but it does have a predilection for the periventricular structures.

7-18. The answer is a. *(Fauci, pp 468-473.)* This patient has morbid obesity (BMI over 40) and has comorbidities of hypertension, diabetes, and osteoarthritis of the knees. Two large meta-analyses have established that bariatric surgery is more effective than nonsurgical therapy for achieving sustained weight loss and controlling comorbid conditions for patients with morbid obesity. Surgical mortality is low (less than 1%) and associated with long-term sustained weight loss of 45 to 65 pounds. Several professional organizations, including the American College of Physicians, now recommend bariatric surgery as the treatment of choice for patients with morbid obesity, especially if they have comorbid conditions and have failed dietary therapy. Controlled trials have established that caloric restriction and physical activity can achieve modest weight reduction, usually on the order of 2% to 8%. A review of commercial weight-loss programs demonstrated that Weight Watchers was the most effective with a sustained weight reduction of 3% at 2 years. A number of medications (sibutramine, orlistat, and phentermine) are FDA approved for weight reduction but have demonstrated only modest effectiveness. Sibutramine is associated with dry mouth and can elevate blood pressure and therefore is not a good choice for this patient. This patient has morbid obesity with comorbid conditions and has failed dietary therapy and exercise program. Therefore his physician should discuss the possibility of bariatric surgery for treatment of his obesity.

7-19. The answer is c. *(Brunicardi, pp 1531-1532.)* Lesions that are solid and enhancing on CT scan should raise the suspicion for a renal cell carcinoma. Because of a high false-negative rate, suspicious lesions should not routinely be biopsied. For renal cell cancers less than 4 cm, a partial nephrectomy can be performed, but for larger lesions, a radical nephrectomy (which includes the kidney, ipsilateral adrenal gland, and perirenal fat) is indicated. Benign kidney lesions include simple cysts, angiomyolipomas, and oncocytomas. Simple cysts do not require further follow-up, but multiple septations or calcifications should increase suspicion for malignancy. Angiomyolipomas can be diagnosed based on appearance on CT scan and do not require removal; larger lesions are at increased risk for hemorrhagic complications. Oncocytomas can be diagnosed only on pathology.

7-20. The answer is d. (*Kaplan, p 20.*) This woman is likely suffering from alcohol dependence, because her child is showing the classic signs of a fetal alcohol syndrome. This syndrome affects approximately one-third of all infants born to women afflicted with alcoholism. Besides the signs this infant has, one can see delayed development, hyperactivity, attention deficits, learning disabilities, intellectual deficits, and seizures in these children.

7-21. The answer is e. (*Rosen, pp 1210-1224. Tintinalli, pp 386-391.*) **D-dimer** is a degradation product produced by plasmin-mediated proteolysis of cross-linked fibrin. There are two types of D-dimer assays. Those with greatest sensitivity are the enzyme-linked immunosorbent assays and the turbidimetric assays. Because of their high negative predictive value, D-dimer levels are typically used to **rule out the diagnosis of PE.** In conjunction with a low pretest probability, a negative D-dimer is predictive of not having a PE. Therefore, in this patient with a high probability of PE (eg, exhibiting dyspnea, chest pain, tachycardia, malignancy), it is likely that the D-dimer will be abnormal.

(a) Arterial blood gas has a very low predictive value in a typical population of patients in whom PE is suspected because they typically have some pulmonary pathology that affects pulmonary gas exchange more than a PE does. Most patients with a PE have a normal PaO_2. (b) Oxygen saturation is rarely depressed and not very useful in the workup of PE. (c) The most common ECG findings are tachycardia and nonspecific ST/T-wave abnormalities. Occasionally, signs of right heart strain are noted. (d) Chest radiographs are usually normal. Twenty-four to seventy-two hours after a PE, atelectasis or a focal infiltrate may be seen. Radiographic findings classically associated with PE are Hampton hump (triangular pleural-based infiltrate) and Westermark sign (dilation of pulmonary vessels proximal to PE with collapse of distal vessels).

7-22. The answer is d. (*Executive Committee for the Asymptomatic Carotid Atherosclerosis Study, pp 1421-1428.*) In a prospective, randomized, multicenter trial involving 1662 patients in a study known as the Asymptomatic Carotid Atherosclerosis Study, patients with asymptomatic carotid artery stenosis causing 60% or greater reduction in diameter and whose general health made them good candidates for elective surgery were found to have a significant reduction in the 5-year risk for ipsilateral stroke with surgery compared with medically treated cohorts (5.1% vs 11.0%). Medically treated patients were treated with aspirin on a daily basis. Warfarin has not been shown to be effective in the management of patients with carotid disease. Angioplasty of carotid stenoses is being performed in some institutions but to date has not replaced surgery as the treatment for high-grade carotid stenoses.

7-23. The answer is a. *(South-Paul, pp 233-248.)* Extra-articular manifestations of RA can be seen at any stage of the disease. Most common are rheumatoid nodules that can occur anywhere on the body, but usually subcutaneously along pressure points. Vasculitis, dry eyes, dyspnea, or cough can all be seen. Cough and dyspnea may signal respiratory interstitial disease. Cardiac, GI, and renal systems are rarely involved. When a neuropathy is present, it is generally because of a compression syndrome, not as an extra-articular manifestation of the disease.

7-24. The answer is b. *(Bieber, pp 31, 831-840.)* While each of the options will provide contraception, only the combination pill fulfills all of her requests. Tubal ligations are permanent sterilization. Progesterone-infused IUDs provide convenient and effective reversible contraception; they usually decrease menstrual flow and do not cause significant weight gain. IUDs, however, are not effective in treating acne or premenstrual dysphoric disorder (PMDD). Progesterone intramuscular injections are associated with weight gain. Condoms do not provide benefits beyond contraception and protection against sexually transmitted infections. The only FDA approved contraceptive pill for PMDD is a drospirenone/ethinyl estradiol combination.

7-25. The answer is e. *(Hay, pp 885-888. Kliegman, pp 2116-2120. McMillan, pp 1750-1758. Rudolph, pp 1594-1600.)* Children who present with symptoms that suggest leukemia with bone marrow failure require a bone marrow biopsy as soon as possible to clarify the diagnosis. Leukemias are the most common childhood malignancy, accounting for about 40% of all malignancies in children less than 15 years of age. Two thousand children a year are diagnosed with acute lymphoblastic leukemia (ALL) in the United States. Most are between the ages of 2 and 6 years; a male predominance is noted. All of the symptoms in the vignette are typically found with leukemia: clinical and laboratory evidence of marrow failure with anemia and thrombocytopenia. The WBC count can be normal, high, or low. Automated systems initially may report blast forms as atypical lymphocytes. A reticulocyte count would reflect lack of marrow response, but is nonspecific. EBV can cause fever and listlessness with lymphadenopathy, but is usually not associated with significant anemia and thrombocytopenia as described here. Haptoglobin may help distinguish hemolytic from nonhemolytic anemia, and an antiplatelet antibody would not explain the anemia.

7-26. The answer is a. (*Mengel, pp 300-306.*) When the history, physical examination, 12-lead ECG, and limited laboratory evaluation are negative, it is appropriate to reassure the patient with palpitations and continue observation. The likely etiology is benign supraventricular or ventricular ectopy. Other tests and consultation would only be indicated if the patient's symptoms are incapacitating or worrisome.

7-27. The answer is a. (*Kaplan p 140.*) This infant is displaying the protest phase of a separation, which occurs approximately 3 days after a young, well-attached child is separated from a parent. The protest phase is characterized by crying, calling, and searching for the parent. If the parent reappears shortly thereafter, before the child enters the despair phase of separation, the anger of the child is evidenced by his or her ambivalent response to the parent's return. This can be seen by the child refusing affection from the parent, turning his or her head away, and wanting to remain with the alternate caregiver. The despair phase, which follows the protest phase, is demonstrated by an air of hopelessness about the child, who even though still attached to the parent, may appear indifferent upon the parent's return. If the separation continues, the child enters the detachment phase, when the bond with the parent has been irreparably severed.

7-28. The answer is c. (*Ropper, p 51.*) A number of spinal cord processes could have produced this evolving paraplegia. Rapid investigation is essential to maximize the likelihood that this young man will recover cord function once the lesion has been treated. Even a reversible lesion left untreated for days or weeks will lead to permanent disability. Magnetic resonance imaging scanning is the best emergent test when available, as it will show compressive lesions as well as processes, such as tumors, inflammation, or infection, which may affect the parenchyma of the spinal cord itself. Vascular lesions, such as spinal cord AVMs, may also be seen on MRI, although spinal angiography is often required to confirm the lesion and guide therapy. Anticoagulation is ill advised, because any one of several processes, such as tumors, vascular malformations, or infections, may have already led to bleeding into the spinal cord or be susceptible to bleeding. The patient in the case history had schistosomiasis.

7-29. The answer is c. (*Katz, p 334.*) Nipple discharge can occur in women with either benign or malignant breast conditions. Approximately 10% to 15% of women with benign breast disease complain of nipple discharge.

However, nipple discharge is present in only about 3% of women with breast malignancies. The most worrisome nipple discharges tend to be spontaneous, unilateral, and persistent. The color of nipple discharge does not differentiate benign from malignant breast conditions. The most common breast disorder associated with a bloody nipple discharge is an intraductal papilloma. However, breast carcinoma must always be ruled out in any patient complaining of a bloody nipple discharge. Sanguineous or serosanguineous nipple discharges can also be seen in women with duct ectasia and fibrocystic breast disease. Women with hyperprolactinemia caused by a pituitary adenoma experience bilateral milky white nipple discharges.

7-30. The answer is e. *(South-Paul, pp 233-248.)* Oral steroids have a strong potential for ulcer formation, and although they may offer temporary relief, would not be indicated for chronic osteoarthritis. Another steroid injection would be of limited benefit, and most recommend no more than two injections per year to avoid hastening of the osteoarthritic process. Ketorolac is not indicated for intra-articular injection. Hyaluronic acid injections have been shown to provide symptomatic relief in osteoarthritis for up to 6 months, but given the malalignment demonstrated in his x-ray, knee replacement would likely be more beneficial. Indications for replacement include poorly controlled pain despite maximal therapy, malalignment, and decreased mobility or ambulation.

7-31. The answer is c. *(Fauci, pp 687-700.)* Chronic lymphocytic leukemia is the most common of all leukemias, with incidence increasing with age. Patients are usually asymptomatic, but may complain of weakness, fatigue, or enlarged lymph nodes. The diagnosis is made by peripheral blood smear, as mature small lymphocytes constitute almost all the white blood cells seen. Smudge cells are often present. No other process produces a lymphocytosis of this morphology and magnitude. The leukemic cells in acute leukemia are immature blast cells that are easily distinguished from the normal-appearing mature lymphocytes of CLL. Both chronic myelogenous leukemia and the leukemoid reaction associated with illness such as TB are associated with increased numbers of a variety of cells of the myeloid series (mature polymorphonuclear leukocytes, metamyelocytes, myelocytes, etc). The peripheral blood is said to resemble a dilute preparation of bone marrow. The presence of basophilia would suggest CML. Infectious mononucleosis would be rare at this age and causes large "atypical" lymphocytes that are easily distinguished from mature lymphocytes on peripheral smear.

7-32. The answer is a. *(Ropper, pp 554-555.)* There are several different grading schemes for astrocytoma, but Kernohan's classification of grades from I (least malignant) to IV (most malignant) is the one most widely used. Glioblastoma multiforme is an older term for the grade IV astrocytoma and is still in general use. This is a highly malignant tumor that develops most often in the cerebral hemispheres. The most malignant tumors usually exhibit areas of necrosis and have a poor prognosis. Survival with glioblastoma multiforme is usually measured in months rather than years. Treatment generally consists of gross total resection and radiation therapy. Survival may be increased to 40 weeks after this combination of therapies, whereas it is on average only 14 weeks after surgery alone. The intravenous medications listed are antineoplastic agents, but they are not effective against this type of tumor. Some chemotherapy has been generally regarded as useful for this type of primary brain tumor including 1,3-bis (2-chloroethyl)-1-nitrosourea (BCNU), which increases survival only marginally.

7-33 to 7-36. The answers are 33-h, 34-c, 35-e, 36-a. *(Kaplan, pp 98-110.)* CNS neurotransmitters include amino acids, biogenic amines, and neuropeptides. There are many other neurotransmitter substances, and many are still poorly understood. This is one of the most exciting areas of current psychiatric research. As more and more knowledge accrues, it becomes possible to develop more specific psychopharmacologic interventions. Glutamic and aspartic acids have excitatory properties. GABA is the principal inhibitory neurotransmitter. The biogenic amines include the catecholamines such as dopamine, norepinephrine, epinephrine, histamine, and the indolamine serotonin. Neuropeptides include β-endorphin, somatostatin, and vasopressin, and substance P. Serotonin is affected primarily by fluoxetine, as it is a serotonin-specific reuptake inhibitor. Norepinephrine is affected by a wide array of the classical antidepressant drugs, as well as some of the newer drugs like mirtazapine. Substance P is known to mediate the perception of pain, and neuropeptide Y has been shown to stimulate the appetite, making it an area of interest for obesity researchers.

7-37. The answer is a. *(Hay, pp 1120-1123. Kliegman, pp 1377-1379, McMillan, pp 511-515. Rudolph, pp 1031-1035.)* Periventricular calcifications are a characteristic finding in infants who have congenital CMV infection. The encephalitic process especially affects the subependymal tissue around the lateral ventricles and thus results in the periventricular deposition of calcium. Calcified tuberculomas, if visible radiographically, are not particularly periventricular; congenital tuberculosis presenting such as the patient described would be extraordinarily unusual. Granulomatous encephalitis caused by congenital toxoplasmosis is associated with scattered and soft-appearing intracranial calcification, and suprasellar calcifications are typical of craniopharyngiomas. Congenital syphilis does not produce intracranial calcifications. The unscientific, but sometimes useful, way of keeping intracranial calcifications caused by CMV differentiated from those caused by toxoplasmosis is to remember that "CMV" has a V in it, as does "periventricular"; "toxoplasmosis" has an X in it, and the lesions associated with it are scattered throughout the "cortex," which also has an X in it.

7-38. The answer is e. (*Rosen, pp 1110-1130.*) This patient is showing signs and symptoms of **CHF**, which is classified as either right- or left-sided. Right-sided heart failure manifests as jugular venous distention, ascites, and peripheral edema. Left-sided heart failure manifests as pulmonary edema or shock. This patient has both as left-sided failure often leads to right-sided failure. Outpatient management for CHF includes a β-blocker to decrease cardiac stress and improve contractility, a loop diuretic to aid in diuresis of excess fluid; and an ACE inhibitor for both BP management and renal-protective effects. Patients should also take a daily aspirin (**b**) for cardiac protection. Calcium channel blockers (**d**) are not specifically indicated for CHF.

7-39. The answer is c. (*Rosen, pp 986-998.*) **PCP** is a commonly seen opportunistic infection in the HIV/AIDS population. It typically presents with mild subjective symptoms of cough and general malaise. Objectively, patients are hypoxic and have a chest radiograph with a bilateral interstitial process. Risk factors include a **CD4 count < 200**. Serum lactate dehydrogenase (LDH) is also considerably higher in AIDS patients with PCP. In fact, greater the elevation in LDH, worse the prognosis. Despite the classic PCP radiograph demonstrating bilateral diffuse interstitial infiltrates, beginning in the perihilar region and extending into a "bat-wing" pattern, the chest radiograph may be normal in up to 30% of patients. In addition to Kaposi sarcoma involvement in the lungs, pulmonary infections, such as tuberculosis, cytomegalovirus, and fungal infections, should be considered.

  Coccidioidomycosis (**a**) is caused by the fungus *C immitis*. The fungus is endemic in the southwestern United States. Conformation of the diagnosis is made through direct observation of the fungus in smear or culture, or through the detection of serum antibodies. The chest radiograph generally reveals mediastinal or hilar adenopathy, pleural effusions, nodules, cavitations, or infiltrates. *Mycobacterium tuberculosis* (**b**) is the causative organism of tuberculosis (TB). Patients can present with chronic cough, hemoptysis, and constitutional symptoms. Because TB can present in a clinically similar fashion as PCP in immunocompromised individuals, TB studies should also be performed on this patient. In classic reactivation TB, pulmonary lesions are located in the posterior segment of the right-upper lobe, apicoposterior segment of the left-upper lobe, and apical segments of the lower lobes. In the presence of HIV or other immunosuppressant disease, lesions are often atypical. Up to 20% of patients who are HIV positive with active disease have normal chest x-ray findings. Radiographic findings consistent with active primary TB are similar to those of lobar pneumonia with ipsilateral hilar adenopathy. *Mycoplasma pneumoniae* (**d**) is a common cause of community-acquired pneumonia in patients under the age of 40. Radiographic findings are variable, but abnormalities are usually more striking than the findings on physical examination. *Haemophilus influenzae* (**e**) is common among patients with COPD, alcoholism, malnutrition, or malignancy.

7-40. The answer is c. (*Hay, pp 582-583. Kleigman, pp 1036-1042. McMillan, pp 1015-1023. Rudolph, pp 844-845.*) Many conditions can be associated with prolonged fever, a limp caused by arthralgia, exanthem, adenopathy, and pharyngitis. Conjunctivitis, however, is suggestive of Kawasaki disease. The fissured lips, although common in Kawasaki disease, could occur after a long period of fever from any cause if the child became dehydrated. The predominance of neutrophils and high ESR are common to all. An increase in platelets within this constellation of symptoms, however, is found typically in Kawasaki disease. Kawasaki disease presents as a picture of prolonged fever, rash, epidermal peeling on the hands and feet (especially around the fingertips), conjunctivitis, lymphadenopathy, fissured lips, oropharyngeal mucosal erythema, and arthralgia or arthritis. The diagnosis is still possible in the absence of one or two of these physical findings. Coronary artery aneurysms can develop, as can aneurysms in other areas. Initial treatment is typically intravenous immunoglobulin (IVIG) and high-dose aspirin. The child will usually defervesce shortly after the infusion. Aspirin is typically kept at a higher dose until the platelet count begins to decrease, and then is continued at a lower dose for several weeks. While bacterial infection is in the differential diagnosis for this patient's presentation and blood cultures are usually part of the evaluation, IV vancomycin should be reserved for a culture-proven susceptible organism resistant to other antibiotics, or as empiric therapy in a critically ill patient.

7-41. The answer is e. (*Fauci, pp 2531-2534.*) This patient has the classic presentation of an intraparenchymal (intracerebral) hemorrhage, that is,

sudden onset of headache with progressive hemiparesis and the development of obtundation caused by brainstem compression. Although approximately 25% of ischemic strokes are associated with headache, a severe and
progressive headache usually indicates intracerebral bleeding. The usual
cause is poorly controlled hypertension, but this patient's compliance with
his antihypertensive regimen, the lack of an S_4 gallop and the absence of
left ventricular hypertrophy militate against this diagnosis. In addition,
hypertensive bleeds are usually in the central structures of the brain (eg,
thalamus, basal ganglia, cerebellum) whereas this patient has a lobar hemorrhage (ie, blood in the parietal lobe). This is the classic presentation of
cerebral amyloid angiopathy, a disease of the elderly associated with con-
gophilic deposits in the cerebral vessels. The vessels are weakened and typically cause recurrent lobar hemorrhages. Rarely is there evidence of
systemic amyloidosis. The prognosis is poor and treatment usually unsuccessful. True CNS vasculitis is usually associated with a chronic or subacute
course and evidence of systemic involvement. Trauma and coagulopathy
are usually associated with fracture or ecchymosis.

7-42 to 7-46. The answers are 42-a, 43-e, 44-b, 45-d, 46-c. (*Reece,
pp 813-815. Cunningham, pp 446-456.*) Fetal heart rate tracings are obtained
in most pregnancies in the United States through the use of electronic fetal
monitoring equipment. Accurate interpretation of these tracings with resul-
tant action to expedite delivery in fetuses threatened by hypoxia has
improved neonatal outcome, although it has had very little effect on the
overall incidence of cerebral palsy, which seems most often to have its etiology remote from the time of labor. Tracing **a** shows a classic hyperstimula-
tion pattern, with a tonic contraction lasting several minutes with distinctly
raised intrauterine pressure and a consequent fall in fetal heart rate. Despite
the increased uterine pressure, there remains good beat-to-beat variability,
which suggests that the fetus is withstanding the stress. Tracing **b** shows
fetal heart rate accelerations occurring spontaneously both before and after
contractions, with good beat-to-beat variability, and is representative of a
very healthy fetus. Tracing **c** shows late decelerations following two consecutive contractions. The baseline variability is significantly reduced. This pattern is caused by uteroplacental insufficiency. Tracing **d** shows variable
decelerations in which the classic V-shaped picture of a variable deceleration
is maintained. Such decelerations are a normal, reflex response to umbilical
cord compression.

Block 8

Answers

8-1. The answer is e. *(Fauci, pp 1619-1628.)* The term "healthcare-associated pneumonia" is used to describe patients with increased risk for drug-resistant etiologies of pneumonia. Residents of long-term care facilities as well as patients with recent antibiotic exposure, recent hospitalization, chronic dialysis, and home wound care are at greater risk of pneumonia from multidrug resistant (MDR) bacteria such as *Pseudomonas aeruginosa,* extended-spectrum beta-lactamase gram-negative bacilli, *Acinetobacter,* and methicillin-resistant *Staphylococcus aureus.* As such, it would be inappropriate to treat this patient in the same manner as a community dweller without risk factors for MDR. Instead of the typical community-acquired pneumonia (CAP) coverage (third-generation cephalosporin and macrolide or a respiratory fluoroquinolone as in answers a, b, and c), the patient should also be empirically treated for the MDR bacteria listed above. The carbapenem and fluoroquinolone would cover potentially resistant gram-negative rods; the glycopeptide (vancomycin is often used) would cover MRSA. Of note, the patient in this vignette has an estimated creatinine clearance of 25 mL/min. Renal dose adjustment of her antibiotics would be appropriate.

8-2. The answer is b. *(Ropper, pp 230-233.)* The red glass test produces two images because the eyes are not moving in concert. That the red image appears to the left indicates that the eye covered by the red glass is not moving to the left as much as the other eye. A convenient way to remember this is simply to assume that the eye is not moving where the red image appears to be. This assumes that the red glass is over the impaired eye and that ocular motor function in the other eye is completely normal. Additionally, the outside image is always the false image. That the patient has pain behind the right eye and that the pupil of this eye reacts less vigorously to light than the pupil of the other eye suggests that the right eye is solely (or at least disproportionately) involved. Since the medial rectus and pupillary constrictor are involved, the lesioned nerve must be CN III.

8-3. The answer is c. *(Kaplan, p 366.)* Lyme disease is characterized by a bull's-eye rash at the site of the tick bite, followed by a flu-like illness which is often short-lived and may go unnoticed. Problems with cognitive functioning and mood changes may be the first complaints seen. These include problems concentrating, irritability, fatigue, and a depressed mood. Treatment consists of a 2- to 3-week course of doxycycline, which is curative about 90% of the time. If the disease is left untreated, 60% of patients will develop a chronic condition.

8-4. The answer is d. *(Ropper, pp 214-215.)* Ischemic optic neuropathy, often called *anterior ischemic optic neuropathy* (AION), is the most common cause of acute monocular blindness. This condition presents as sudden, painless loss of vision in one eye. Symptoms may progress over several days, and the visual loss is permanent. The visual field defect is typically an inferior altitudinal defect, with involvement of central vision and a consequent loss of acuity. In up to one-third of patients, the opposite eye may become involved soon afterward. Hypertension and diabetes mellitus appear to be risk factors, as for most small-vessel disease. The responsible arterial occlusion is of the posterior ciliary artery, a branch of the ophthalmic artery, which supplies the optic nerve. Typically, this condition is not associated with carotid artery disease. Giant cell arteritis (temporal arteritis) needs to be excluded, because it can be treated with steroids.

8-5. The answer is e. *(Rosen, pp 2069-2074.)* Acetaminophen is one of the most commonly used analgesic-antipyretic medications and causes more hospitalizations after overdose than by any other pharmaceutical agent. Risk of hepatotoxicity is best established by plotting the acetaminophen concentration on the acetaminophen nomogram. Acetaminophen concentration must be measured between 4 and 24 hours after ingestion and then plotted on the nomogram. Patients with acetaminophen concentrations on or above the treatment line should be treated. This patient has a 4-hour serum acetaminophen concentration of 350 μg/mL. According to the nomogram, at 4 hours any concentration above 200 μg/mL should be treated. Therefore, the **patient should be started on NAC** and **admitted to the hospital.** During her admission, she should be evaluated by a psychiatrist regarding her attempted suicide.

The patient is at risk for acetaminophen toxicity and meets criteria for treatment with NAC. Without treatment with NAC, she is at risk of developing liver failure and possible death. The patient is in first phase of an acetaminophen poisoning. This phase usually lasts 0.5 to 24 hours. Patients are usually asymptomatic or exhibit findings such as nausea, vomiting, anorexia, malaise, and diaphoresis.

8-6. The answer is c. *(Rosen, p 2169.)* Patients with initial flu-like symptoms **from the same household** who were exposed to combustion products (ie, from a home generator) are at risk for **carbon monoxide (CO) poisoning.** CO binds to hemoglobin with greater affinity than oxygen and shifts the oxygen-hemoglobin dissociation curve to the left, thus decreasing oxygen release. Clinically, patients with mild CO toxicity present with flu-like symptoms, nausea, and vomiting, which progresses to chest pain, dyspnea, confusion, seizures, dysrhythmias, and coma. CO level can be obtained by a **carboxyhemoglobin level** from blood. CO poisoning is treated with *oxygen* and, if severe, with **hyperbaric oxygen** therapy.

An important clue to the diagnosis is the development of similar symptoms in the patient and her husband at the same time. While it is important to consider ordering a WBC count **(a)**, a head CT scan **(b)**, and an LP **(d)** for evaluation of the symptoms, think CO poisoning when there are multiple patients with the same symptoms in the setting of exposure to combustible products. It is not appropriate to do nothing **(e)** since the patient is clearly in need of medical attention.

8-7. The answer is a. *(Greenfield, pp 442-444; Moore, pp 811-814.)* If the patient is too unstable to perform a definitive repair, placement of a catheter into the proximal ureter is an acceptable alternative that will allow reconstruction to be performed later. Suction drainage adjacent to the injured segment alone is inadequate. If time and the patient's condition permit, primary ureteral reconstruction should be carried out. In the middle third of the ureter, this will usually consist of ureteroureterostomy (primary anastamosis) using absorbable sutures over a stent. If the injury involves the upper third, ureteropyeloplasty may be necessary. In the lower third, ureteral implantation into the bladder using a tunneling technique is preferred. The creation of a watertight seal is difficult and nephrectomy may be required if the injury occurs during a procedure in which a vascular prosthesis is being implanted (eg, an aortic reconstructive procedure) and contamination of the foreign body by urine must be avoided.

8-8. The answer is d. *(Speroff, pp 345-350. Adashi, pp 1008-1015.)* Delayed puberty is a rare condition, usually differentiated into hyper-gonadotropic (high FSH and LH levels) hypogonadism or hypogonadotropic (low FSH and LH) hypogonadism. The most common cause of hypergonadotropic hypogonadism is gonadal dysgenesis (ie, the 45,X Turner syndrome). Hypogonadotropic hypogonadism can be seen in patients with hypothalamic-pituitary or constitutional delays in development. Kallmann syndrome presents with amenorrhea, infantile sexual development, low gonadotropins, normal female karyotype, and anosmia (the inability to perceive odors). In addition to these conditions, many other types of medical and nutritional problems can lead to this type of delayed development (eg, malabsorption, diabetes, regional ileitis, and other chronic illness). Congenital adrenal hyperplasia leads to early pubertal development, although in girls the development is not isosexual (not of the expected sex) and would therefore include hirsutism, clitoromegaly, and other signs of virilization. Complete Müllerian agenesis is a condition in which the Müllerian ducts either fail to develop or regress early in fetal life. These patients have a blind vaginal pouch and no upper vagina, cervix, or uterus, and they present with primary amenorrhea. However, because ovarian development is not affected, secondary sexual characteristics develop normally despite the absence of menarche, and gonadotropin levels are normal. The McCune-Albright syndrome involves the constellation of precocious puberty, café au lait spots, and polyostotic fibrous dysplasia.

8-9. The answer is c. *(Jacobson, pp 61, 187.)* Schizotypal personality disorder, a cluster A disorder, is characterized by acute discomfort in close relationships, cognitive and perceptual distortions, and eccentric behavior beginning in early adulthood and present in a variety of contexts. Individuals with schizoid personality disorder do not present with the magical thinking, oddity, unusual perceptions, and odd appearance typical of schizotypal individuals. In schizophrenia, psychotic symptoms are much more prolonged and severe. Avoidant individuals avoid social interaction out of shyness and fear of rejection and not out of disinterest or suspiciousness. In autism, social interactions are more severely impaired and stereotyped behaviors are usually present.

8-10. The answer is e. *(Mengel, pp 376-383.)* In men with urinary symptoms and a normal urinary tract, cystitis, and pyelonephritis are uncommon. Urethritis would be unlikely to cause this systemic illness. The patient described above has acute bacterial prostatitis. Acute prostatitis is most commonly seen in 30- to 50-year-old men, and symptoms include frequency, urgency, and back pain. The patient generally appears acutely ill, and has pyuria. The prostate examination would reveal a boggy, tender, and warm prostate.

8-11. The answer is c. *(Fauci, pp 2711-2712)* This patient meets the diagnostic criteria for generalized anxiety disorder (GAD). GAD is characterized by excessive anxiety occurring at least half the time for a minimum of six months and associated with three or more of the following: restlessness, fatigue, difficulty concentrating, irritability, muscle tension, or sleep disturbance. In addition, the symptoms must result in significant impairment and must not be due to another psychiatric disease, substance abuse or medical conditions such as hyperthyroidism. This disorder is common and occurs in up to 5% of patients seen in primary care offices. Many of these patients have additional psychiatric disease such as depression. Cognitive behavioral therapy and treatment with tricyclic antidepressants or selective serotonin reuptake inhibitors are often beneficial in relieving symptoms, which tend to be chronic. Benzodiazepines often improve symptoms, but may result in dependence. Hyperthyroidism would be associated with symptoms (heat intolerance, tremor) and signs (tachycardia, goiter) of this disorder. Hyperparathyroidism causes depression more often than anxiety and should cause hypercalcemia on the chemistry panel. Sleep apnea would cause abnormal daytime somnolence as its cardinal symptom. This patient's difficulty concentrating is a manifestation of her anxiety disorder; dementia would be very uncommon in a 32 year old.

8-12. The answer is a. (*Hay, pp 607-608. Kliegman, pp 1555-1557. McMillan, pp 371-372. Rudolph, p 1402.*) A history of nonbilious vomiting for 10 days in a child of this age who does not look ill points to infantile hypertrophic pyloric stenosis as the most likely diagnosis; surgical consultation for a likely pyloromyotomy is indicated. The ultrasound in the question demonstrates the thickened pylorus. The incidence of this condition in infants is between 1:200 and 1:750, with males affected more often than females. Although there is no specific pattern of inheritance, a familial incidence has been observed in about 15% of patients. Information about predisposing ancestry is conflicting, as are data concerning the assertion of a firstborn predilection. Metabolic alkalosis with low serum potassium and chloride levels is frequently seen in pyloric stenosis as a result of loss of gastric contents from vomiting. A child with a small-bowel obstruction (who may require an upper GI with small-bowel follow through to help diagnose the point of obstruction) should develop bilious emesis and should not look well 10 days into the illness; similarly, a child with intussusception (who requires an air contrast enema, which is both diagnostic and perhaps therapeutic) would be markedly ill at this point. Gastroenteritis (IV fluids alone to maintain hydration) does not usually last for 10 days. A brain tumor causing increased intracranial pressure could present with isolated emesis, but should show other symptoms such as irritability and somnolence.

8-13. The answer is e. (*Ropper, pp 984-988.*) This woman was at risk for Wernicke encephalopathy. She should have received supplemental thiamine for at least 3 days, even though this would not have prevented the cognitive deterioration that she exhibited. There was no indication for using a neuroleptic (eg, haloperidol, chlorpromazine, or prochlorperazine), even though her alcohol and benzodiazepine use placed her at risk for developing a withdrawal psychosis. The anticholinergic trihexyphenidyl would not be appropriate as either a neuroleptic or an antiepileptic.

8-14. The answer is c. (*Mengel, pp 313-320.*) Eighty percent of ovarian masses in girls younger than 15 years are malignant. Because of the high potential for malignancy, any adnexal mass should be evaluated by transvaginal ultrasound and referral for surgical removal. In many women of childbearing years, adnexal masses are commonly cysts. If the pain is not acute or recurrent, palpable cysts less than 6 cm in size may be monitored with repeat pelvic examination. Ultrasound is reserved for those masses that do not resolve, or those that increase in size. CT and MRI may be useful in some cases, but the ultrasound is the best first test.

8-15. The answer is e. (*Townsend, pp 486-487.*) Emergency measures to reduce intracranial pressure include hyperventilation, mannitol infusion, and elevation of the head of the bed (reverse Trendelenburg position). However, in the face of inadequate volume resuscitation, osmotic diuresis with mannitol and placement of the patient in reverse Trendelenburg may exacerbate the patient's hypotension. CT scanning should be performed as soon as possible along with neurosurgical evaluation in order to determine the need for operative drainage or decompression.

8-16. The answer is e. (*Tintinalli, pp 193-194.*) This ECG shows **third-degree, or complete AV block**. Note that there is **no relationship between the P waves and QRS complexes.** The P waves occur regularly, but since there is no AV conduction, the ventricles do not respond to the P waves. An escape pacemaker at a rate slower than the atrial rate drives the ventricles, producing regular QRS complexes independent of the P waves.

In contrast, normal sinus rhythm **(a)** has a rate between 60 and 100 beats per minute with every P wave followed immediately by a QRS complex (1:1 conduction). First-degree AV block **(b)** has a PR interval greater than 0.20 seconds. Every P wave is still followed by a QRS complex (1:1 conduction). Second-degree Mobitz I (Wenckebach) AV block **(c)** occurs when there is a progressive delay in AV conduction, manifested by a gradually increasing PR interval, followed by a dropped QRS complex. The pattern then spontaneously repeats. Second-degree Mobitz II AV block **(d)** occurs when there is a constant delay in AV conduction (prolonged PR interval), followed by a dropped QRS complex. It is important to recognize these distinct dysrhythmias as their etiologies are different and subtle treatment differences exist.

8-17. The answer is d. *(Ransom, p 52.)* Syphilis is a chronic disease produced by the spirochete *Treponema pallidum*. Because of the spirochete's extreme thinness, it is difficult to detect by light microscopy; therefore, spirochetes are diagnosed by use of a specially adapted technique known as dark-field microscopy. Clinically, syphilis is divided into primary, secondary, and tertiary (or late) stages. In primary syphilis a hard chancre develops. This is a painless ulcer with an indurated base that is usually found on the vulva, vagina, or cervix. Secondary syphilis is the result of hematogenous dissemination of the spirochetes and thus is a systemic disease. There are a number of systemic symptoms depending on the major organs involved. The classic rash of secondary syphilis is red macules and papules over the palms of the hands and the soles of the feet. The manifestations of late syphilis include optic atrophy, tabes dorsalis, generalized paresis, aortic aneurysm, and gummas of the skin and bones.

8-18. The answer is e. *(American Academy of Family Physicians, 2008.)* Of the interventions listed above, only prescribing folic acid has been shown to be beneficial prior to pregnancy. It will decrease the chance of neural tube defects in the baby. The other interventions should be done early in the pregnancy to ensure good pregnancy outcome.

8-19. The answer is d. *(Brunicardi, pp 1447-1448.)* The patient has tertiary hyperparathyroidism, which is manifested by persistent hypercalcemia secondary to autonomous parathyroid function after renal transplantation. Treatment is total parathyroidectomy with autotransplantation or subtotal parathyroidectomy. The imaging modalities described would be more appropriate in the workup of primary hyperparathyroidism—24-hour urinary calcium levels are low in familial hypercalciuric hypercalcemia. Ultrasound, sestamibi scintigraphy, and CT scanning are all modalities that can be utilized to identify a parathyroid adenoma preoperatively.

8-20. The answer is e. *(Fauci, pp 158-162.)* This patient has postoperative delirium, characterized by confusion and agitation that develops abruptly. Frequently the level of consciousness fluctuates. Postoperative delirium is common in the elderly. Males are affected more commonly than females. Delirium occurs more frequently in elderly patients with preexisting dementia, history of alcohol abuse, and memory impairment. Persons with postoperative delirium should receive a careful history that includes medication review, a physical examination, and laboratory testing. Laboratory testing should be directed toward excluding electrolyte disturbance, infection, and hypoxemia. The most common treatable causes of delirium are related to medications and electrolyte disturbances. Medicines with anticholinergic and sedating property should be avoided. Commonly prescribed drugs with anticholinergic properties include diphenhydramine, tricyclic antidepressants, oxybutynin, and H_2 blocking agents. Management of postoperative delirium includes looking for underlying precipitating factors, correcting electrolyte disturbances, discontinuing aggravating medications, removing indwelling devices, avoiding physical or pharmacologic restraints, early mobilization, and the use the orienting stimuli such as clocks and calendars. Postoperative delirium is a serious condition and has been associated with an increased mortality, prolonged hospital stay, and chance of nursing home placement after hospitalization.

Structural central nervous system disease is an uncommon cause of postoperative delirium; so CT scanning would not be the first test ordered. Pulmonary embolism can cause delirium by causing hypoxia; since this patient's oxygen saturation is normal, lung scan would not be indicated. Infection can cause postoperative delirium, but this patient's normal temperature and white blood cell count militate against an infectious cause. Restraints and benzodiazepines often make delirium worse. If pharmacotherapy is required, haloperidol or an atypical antipsychotic is usually the first choice.

8-21. The answer is a. (*Kaplan, pp 81-85.*) Positron emission tomography (PET) scan has consistently demonstrated a decrease in blood flow and metabolism in the frontal lobe of depressed patients. Most studies have found bilateral rather than unilateral deficits and equivalent decreases in several types of depression (unipolar, bipolar, associated with OCD). Cortical atrophy and subcortical infarcts are associated, respectively, with Alzheimer disease and multi-infarct dementia. Atrophy of the caudate is characteristic of Huntington's disease. In major depression, the REM sleep latency (the period of time between falling asleep and the first period of REM sleep) is shortened, not prolonged.

8-22. The answer is c. (*Lee, pp 143-148.*) Both type 1 and type 2 Chiari malformations are primarily abnormalities of hindbrain development. With the type 1, or adult, abnormality, the cerebellar tonsils extend below the foramen magnum. Affected persons do not usually become symptomatic until they are adults, and then the symptoms are largely referable to the cerebellum. With the type 2 malformation, cerebellar anatomy is usually much more deranged, and the cerebellar vermis lies well below the foramen magnum. Type 2 malformations most often become symptomatic at birth or during infancy and may produce hydrocephalus with retardation.

8-23 to 8-24. The answers are 23-b, 24-e. *(Kaplan, p 803.)* The essential feature of narcissistic personality disorder is a pervasive pattern of grandiosity, need for admiration, and lack of empathy that begins by early adulthood. Individuals with this disorder overestimate their abilities, inflate their accomplishments, and expect others to share the unrealistic opinion they have of themselves. They believe they are special and unique and attribute special qualities to those with whom they associate. When they do not receive the admiration they think they deserve, people with narcissistic personality react with anger and devaluation. The prevalence of the disorder is estimated at less than 1% of the general population, and 50% to 75% of those diagnosed with narcissistic personality are males. In contrast with their outward appearance, individuals with this disorder have a very vulnerable sense of self. Criticism leaves them feeling degraded and hollow. Narcissistic traits are common in adolescence, but most individuals do not progress to develop narcissistic personality disorder. Treatment of narcissistic personality disorder is extremely difficult and requires a tactful therapist who can make confrontations, but do it gently. Forming an alliance with these patients can be very difficult. Medications do not work for this disorder. Psychoanalysis would be too intense for a patient with this disorder, and the abstinent stance would quickly drive the patient from therapy. Likewise, group therapy with a heterogeneous group would likely enrage a narcissist, who would be unable to take criticism from the other group members. Sometimes homogeneous groups of patients (a group with all narcissists, for example) might be able to work together therapeutically because it would help them understand their own maladaptive patterns as they watch others' behaviors.

8-25. The answer is b. *(Brunicardi, pp 276-281.)* A surgeon is frequently asked to evaluate patients who are receiving systemic chemotherapy. Most complications of chemotherapy do not require surgical therapy. Perirectal abscesses are more common in these immunosuppressed patients. GI bleeding occurs secondary to mucosal irritation and thrombocytopenia. Pancreatitis is uncommon, but is associated with L-asparaginase use. Up to 20% of patients treated with floxuridine by continuous hepatic artery infusion develop some degree of inflammation and obstruction of the bile duct.

Systemic chemotherapy does not increase the likelihood of acute cholecystitis, appendicitis, incarcerated femoral hernia, or diverticulitis.

8-26. The answer is b. *(Kaplan, pp 766-767.)* The child in the question is experiencing episodes of sleep terror disorder, a dyssomnia characterized by sudden partial arousal accompanied by piercing screams, motor agitation, disorientation, and autonomic arousal. The episodes take place during the transition from deep sleep to REM sleep. Children do not report nightmares (which would be associated with REM sleep) and do not have any memory of the episodes the next day. Sleep terrors occur in 3% of children and 1% of adults. Although specific treatment for this disorder is seldom required, in rare cases it is necessary. Diazepam (Valium) in small doses at bedtime improves the condition and sometimes completely eliminates the attacks.

8-27. The answer is a. *(Beckmann, pp 129-131. Cunningham, pp 1241-1245.)* This patient is exhibiting classic symptoms of postpartum depression. Postpartum depression develops in about 8% to 15% of women and generally is characterized by an onset about 2 weeks to 12 months postdelivery and an average duration of 3 to 14 months. Women with postpartum depression have the following symptoms: irritability, labile mood, difficulty sleeping, phobias, and anxiety. About 50% of women experience postpartum blues, or maternity blues, within 3 to 6 days after delivering. This mood disturbance is thought to be precipitated by progesterone withdrawal following delivery and usually resolves in 10 days. Maternity blues is characterized by mild insomnia, tearfulness, fatigue, irritability, poor concentration, and depressed affect. Postpartum psychosis usually has its onset within a few days of delivery and is characterized by confusion, disorientation, and loss of touch with reality. Postpartum psychosis is very rare and occurs in only 1 to 4 in 1000 births. Bipolar disorder or manic-depressive illness is a psychiatric disorder characterized by episodes of depression followed by mania.

8-28. The answer is b. *(Mengel, pp 219-223.)* There are several medications that can cause hematuria. They include penicillins, cephalosporins, sulfonamides, phenytoin, cyclophosphamide, mitotane, anticoagulants, and nitrofurantoin. Ibuprofen may cause kidney problems, but hematuria is not one of them.

8-29. The answer is c. *(Hay, p 485. Kliegman, pp 1754-1756. McMillan, pp 1493-1494. Rudolph, p 1944.)* Suppurative infection of the chain of lymph nodes between the posterior pharyngeal wall and the prevertebral fascia leads to retropharyngeal abscesses. The most common causative organisms are *S aureus,* group A β-hemolytic streptococci, and oral anaerobes. Presenting signs and symptoms include a history of pharyngitis, abrupt onset of fever with severe sore throat, refusal of food, drooling, and muffled or noisy breathing. A bulge in the posterior pharyngeal wall is diagnostic, as are radiographs of the lateral neck that reveal the retropharyngeal mass (the radiograph in the question demonstrates thickening of the pre-vertebral space). Palpation (with adequate provision for emergency control of the airway in case of rupture) reveals a fluctuant mass. Treatment should include incision and drainage if fluctuance is present. All of the wrong answers listed would delay definitive treatment and/or might be life threatening.

8-30. The answer is c. *(Ropper, pp 698-699.)* Based on the results of the North American Symptomatic Carotid Endarterectomy Trial (NASCET), it is known that carotid endarterectomy can reduce the risk of stroke in patients with symptomatic stenosis by 70% or more. The risk of ipsilateral stroke was reduced from 26% in the medically treated group to 9% in the surgically treated group. Carotid endarterectomy should be offered to all eligible patients with symptomatic disease of the internal carotid artery. Carotid angioplasty with stenting is an alternative for management of these patients. However, it is less established than endarterectomy. Angioplasty without stenting is not indicated. Extracranial–intracranial bypass has been tried unsuccessfully, although it may still play a role for certain patients with inaccessible lesions or hypoperfusion in the setting of complete occlusions. Aspirin would be appropriate after endarterectomy.

8-31. The answer is b. *(Tintinalli, pp 252-255.)* This patient is in **neurogenic shock.** He suffered an acute cervical spine injury after his fall onto rocks and has **hypotension** and **bradycardia.** The pathophysiology behind neurogenic shock is still under investigation but it's thought to be partially caused by **disrupted sympathetic outflow tracts** and **unopposed vagal tone.** Note that all other forms of shock attempt to compensate for hypotension with tachycardia. Neurogenic shock lacks sympathetic innervation; therefore, bradycardia results. Given that this is a trauma patient, all other sources for hypotension must be ruled out. He should be treated with cervical spine immobilization and IV fluids. Pressors may be needed if hypotension does not respond to fluids or fluid overload becomes a concern.

Hypovolemic shock (**a**) occurs when there is inadequate volume in the circulatory system, resulting in poor oxygen delivery to the tissues. Cardiogenic shock (**c**) is caused by decreased cardiac output producing inadequate

tissue perfusion. Anaphylactic shock (d) is a severe systemic hypersensitivity reaction resulting in hypotension and airway compromise. Septic shock
(e) is a clinical syndrome of hypoperfusion, hypotension, or multiorgan
dysfunction caused by infection.

8-32. The answer is d. (*McPhee, pp 191-192*) The clinical features most
suggestive of group A β-hemolytic streptococcal pharyngitis are fever, tender
anterior cervical adenopathy, lack of cough, and a pharyngotonsillar exudates. These four features are called the Centor criteria, and when present,
strongly suggest infection, and the most cost effective approach is to treat
without performing laboratory testing. When three of the four criteria are
present, the laboratory sensitivity of a rapid antigen test exceeds 90%. When
only one criterion is present, strep is unlikely. Marked adenopathy and a
shaggy white-purple tonsillar exudates is more suggestive of mononucleosis.

8-33. The answer is e. (*Brunicardi, pp 796-797.*) Atherosclerotic occlusion
of the subclavian artery proximal to the vertebral artery is the anatomic situation that results in the subclavian steal syndrome. On being subjected to
exercise, the involved extremity (usually the left, which is more prone to
atherosclerosis because of anatomic differences) develops relative ischemia,
which gives rise to reversal of flow through the vertebral artery with consequent diminished flow to the brain. The upper extremity symptom is intermittent claudication. Venous occlusive disease is not a feature of the
syndrome. The operative procedure for treating the subclavian steal syndrome consists of delivering blood to the extremity by creating either a
carotid-subclavian bypass or a subclavian-carotid transposition. Dilatation
and stenting of the artery by endovascular techniques is effective as well.

8-34. The answer is b. (*Fauci, pp 564-565.*) Evaluation of a breast nodule
should determine whether the patient has a true mass or prominent physiologic glandular tissue. The next step is to determine whether the dominant mass represents a cyst, a benign solid mass, or cancer. Worrisome
characteristics of this patient's mass include irregular borders, size larger
than 1 cm, and location in the upper outer quadrant of the breast. Her age
(> 35) also places her at slightly higher risk. Therefore, repeat imaging
including mammogram and ultrasound is warranted. Even if the mammogram is negative, a noncystic mass on ultrasound should be examined by a
breast surgeon or a comprehensive breast radiologist and biopsy performed. Six months is too long to wait for reevaluation. In a younger
woman (< 35), repeat examination after the next menstrual cycle might be

warranted (ie, < 1-month reevaluation). To assume breast changes are benign without further investigation is not appropriate. CT scanning does not provide useful information in the evaluation of palpable breast mass.

8-35. The answer is c. (*Cunningham, pp 374-382, 882-890.*) Patients at 41 to 42 weeks gestation with good dating criteria and a favorable cervix should undergo induction of labor. If the cervix is unfavorable, fetal well-being should be assessed prior to allowing the pregnancy to continue. Patient self-assessment by measurement of fetal kick counts, NST, contraction stress testing, and fetal BPP may be used to assess fetal well-being. The BPP allows assessment of the fetal heart rate tracing and the amniotic fluid level, which in this case is the next best step in the management of this patient. Induction of labor is recommended at 42 weeks regardless of the favorability of the cervix because of the increased risk of perinatal morbidity after that gestational age. As noted above, it is not recommended to perform an elective section without a trial of labor because of the risks of major surgery.

8-36. The answer is d. (*Kaplan, pp 929-930.*) Supportive psychotherapy is characterized by an emphasis on the nurturing, caring role of the therapist and a focus on current reality. Although insight-oriented strategies such as interpretations can be used, they are not the main therapeutic instruments. Supportive psychotherapy aims to foster and maintain a positive transference all the time in order to provide the patient with a consistently safe and secure atmosphere. Consolation, advice, reality testing, environmental manipulation, reassurance, and encouragement are strategies commonly used in supportive psychotherapy.

8-37. The answer is a. (*Katz, pp 427-428, 588-590, 782-783.*) Vulvar vestibulitis is a syndrome of unknown etiology. To make the diagnosis of this disorder, the following three findings must be present: (1) severe pain on vestibular touch or attempted vaginal entry, (2) tenderness to pressure localized within the vulvar vestibule, and (3) visible findings confined to vulvar erythema of various degrees. To treat vulvar vestibulitis, the first step is to avoid tight clothing, tampons, hot tubs, and soaps, which can all act as vulvar irritants. If this fails, topical treatments include lidocaine, estrogen, and steroids. Tricyclic antidepressants and intralesional interferon injections have also been used. For women refractory to medical therapy, surgical excision of the vestibular mucosa may be helpful. Valtrex (valacyclovir) is an antiviral medication used in the treatment of genital herpes and is not indicated for vulvar vestibulitis. Contact dermatitis is an inflammation and irritation of the vulvar skin caused by a chemical irritant. The vulvar skin is usually red, swollen, and inflamed and may become weeping and eczemoid. Women with a contact dermatitis usually experience chronic vulvar tenderness, burning, and itching that can occur even when they are not engaging in intercourse. Atrophic vaginitis is a thinning and ulceration of the vaginal mucosa that occurs as a result of hypoestrogenism; thus this condition is usually seen in postmenopausal women not on hormone replacement therapy. Lichen sclerosus is another atrophic condition of the vulva. It is characterized by diffuse, thin whitish epithelial areas on the labia majora, minora, clitoris, and perineum. In severe cases, it may be difficult to identify normal anatomic landmarks. The most common symptom of lichen sclerosus is chronic vulvar pruritus. Vulvar intraepithelial neoplasia (VIN) are precancerous lesions of the vulva that have a tendency to progress to frank cancer. Women with VIN complain of vulvar pruritus, chronic irritation, and raised lesions. These lesions are most commonly located along the posterior vulva and in the perineal body and have a whitish cast and rough texture.

8-38. The answer is b. (*Ropper, pp 717-721.*) The history of a sudden-onset severe headache is very concerning for subarachnoid hemorrhage. Additionally, this patient is in the peak age range for a ruptured cerebral aneurysm. In suspected subarachnoid hemorrhage, CT will detect blood locally or diffusely in more than 90% of cases. However, if no blood is seen, the physician should proceed to a lumbar puncture. Elevated CSF RBCs, xanthochromia, and increased opening pressure all may be caused by subarachnoid hemorrhage. A cerebral angiogram could diagnose the etiology of a subarachnoid hemorrhage, such as an aneurysm; however, it is a more invasive test and should not be done without first attempting to confirm the diagnosis with less risky tests. An MRI is unlikely to give new useful information in this case. Zolmitriptan is a treatment for migraines. This patient's history is not typical for a migraine.

8-39. The answer is d. (*Beckmann, pp 362-364. Speroff, pp 553-560.*) The administration of high-dose estrogen therapy is the preferred way to manage this patient. In women who have suffered heavy and acute bleeding attributed to anovulation, 25 mg of conjugated estrogen can be administered every 4 hours until the bleeding abates. The estrogen will help stop the bleeding by building up the endometrium and stimulating clotting at the capillary level. Since the bleeding is heavy and acute, a D&C will not help stop the bleeding, because the lining is already thinned and atrophic.

In older women, a D&C might be helpful in obtaining tissue for pathology to rule out endometrial cancer. In this young patient who is resuscitated and stabilized with intravenous fluids, there is no indication for a blood transfusion as long as the bleeding abates. Iron therapy alone would not be adequate for this patient; the bleeding must be stopped first. Antiprostaglandins have no role in curtailing hemorrhage in a woman suffering from anovulation. They have been used with some success in ovulatory women who have heavy cycles or in women with menorrhagia caused by use of the intrauterine device. It is thought that prostaglandin synthetase inhibitors reduce the amount of bleeding by promoting vasoconstriction and platelet aggregation.

8-40 to 8-43. The answers are 40-i, 41-f, 42-e, 43-d. (*Hay, pp 23, 506-507, 536, 1106-1108, 1044. Kliegman, pp 721, 726, 750-752, 1773-1777, 1783-1784. McMillan, pp 212, 313-314, 699-700, 1391-1394, 2492. Rudolph, pp 89, 148-151, 186, 191, 1984-1985.*) Infants with upper brachial plexus injury (cervical nerves 3, 4, 5) can also have ipsilateral phrenic nerve paralysis. These infants can present with labored, irregular breathings and cyanosis; the injury is usually unilateral. Confirmation of the diagnosis is made with ultrasound or fluoroscopy which confirms "seesaw" movements during respiration of the two sides of the diaphragm.

Pneumothorax occurs with a frequency of about 1% to 2% of births, but they are rarely symptomatic. Incidence is higher in infants born with meconium-stained fluid, and the chest radiograph is as that described. Transillumination may assist in the diagnosis while awaiting radiograph; immediate treatment for infants with significant distress is with a 23-guage butterfly needle attached to a stopcock and removal of the air. For those without significant distress and who are not on high levels of ambient oxygen, 100% oxygen therapy can assist in nitrogen washout.

Primary pulmonary hypoplasia (Potter sequence) includes a dysmorphic child (widely spaced eyes, low set ears, broad nose, receding chin, limb abnormalities) and bilateral renal agenesis, which leads to oligohydramnios. These infants have immediate respiratory distress; the condition is not compatible with life.

Bronchiolitis is a very common viral infection most often caused by respiratory syncytial virus. It is most often seen in the winter months with symptoms of wheezing, hypoxia, and respiratory distress seen in younger children; often an older sibling has milder, upper respiratory symptoms. Premature infants, infants with congenital heart disease, infants with a variety of lung disorders, and infants with immune system defects are at higher risk of severe complications. Diagnosis is made by clinical history and/or detection of the viral antigen in nasal secretions; treatment is supportive.

8-44 to 8-46. The answers are 44-a, 45-b, 46-e. *(Fauci, pp 225-228, 1010-1019, 1611-1619.)* The 32-year-old male has signs and symptoms of chronic tuberculosis. The disease presents with productive cough, hemoptysis, and weight loss. Night sweats are particularly characteristic of tuberculosis. Chronic cavitary disease usually involves the upper lobes.

The woman who is a heavy cigarette smoker is most likely to have a primary lung tumor. The symptom of hemoptysis in association with weight loss and loss of appetite is particularly concerning. A pulmonary nodule greater than 3 cm is most often malignant, and the shaggy border of the lesion also suggests malignancy. Metastases to the lung are more sharply defined and are usually multiple.

Asbestosis is a risk for those such as construction workers, shipbuilders, and plumbers who may have long-standing history of exposure to asbestos-containing materials. Symptoms are usually subtle and include an annoying dry cough and dyspnea on exertion. Asbestosis on chest x-ray produces a linear interstitial process at the lung bases. Pleural fibrosis and pleural plaques may also be noted, especially on CT scan.

Bibliography

Adashi EY, Rock JA, Rosenwaks Z (eds). *Reproductive Endocrinology, Surgery, and Technology,* Vols 1 and 2. Philadelphia, PA: Lippincott-Raven; 1996.

Advisory Committee on Immunization Practices. Recommended adult immunization schedule: United States, October 2007-September 2008. *Ann Intern Med.* 2007a;147:725-729.

American Academy of Family Physicians, 2008. AAFP Summary of Recommendations for Clinical Preventive Services Tool. Available at http://www.aafp.org/online/en/home/clinical/exam.html. Accessed 12/15/2008.

American College of Obstetricians and Gynecologists. *Circumcision.* Committee Opinion 260, October 2001.

American College of Obstetricians and Gynecologists. *Guidelines for Women's Health Care: A Resource Manual.* 3rd ed. Washington, D.C.: ACOG: 2007.

Aminoff MJ (ed). *Neurology and General Medicine.* 4th ed. Philadelphia, PA: Churchill Livingstone; 2008.

Beckmann CRB, Ling FW, Smith RP, et al (eds). *Obstetrics and Gynecology.* 5th ed. Philadelphia, PA: Lippincott, Williams & Wilkins; 2006.

Bieber EJ, Sanfilippo JS, Horowitz IR. *Clinical Gynecology.* Philadelphia, PA: Churchill-Livingstone Elsevier; 2006.

Brennan T, Blank L, Cohen J, et al. Medical professionalism in the new millennium: A physician charter. *Ann Intern Med.* 2002;136:243-246.

Brunicardi FC, Andersen DK, Billiar TR, et al (eds). *Schwartz's Principles of Surgery.* 8th ed. New York, NY: McGraw-Hill; 2005.

Cunningham FG, Leveno KJ, Bloom SL, et al (eds). *Williams Obstetrics.* 22nd ed. New York, NY: McGraw-Hill; 2005.

DiSaia PJ, Creasman WT (eds). *Clinical Gynecologic Oncology.* 7th ed. St. Louis, MO: Mosby; 2007.

Executive Committee for the Asymptomatic Carotid Atherosclerosis Study, Endarterectomy for asymptomatic carotid artery stenosis. *JAMA.* 1995;273: 1421-1428.

Fauci AS, Braunwald E, Kasper DL, et al (eds). *Harrison's Principles of Internal Medicine.* 17th ed. New York, NY: McGraw-Hill; 2008.

Fleischer G, Ludwig S. *Textbook of Pediatric Emergency Medicine.* 5th ed. Philadelphia, PA: Lippincott, Williams & Wilkins; 2005.

Greenfield LJ, Lillemoe KD, Mulholland MW, et al (eds). *Surgery: Scientific Principles and Practice.* 4th ed. Philadelphia, PA: Lippincott-Raven; 2005.

Hay WW, Levin MJ, Sondheimer JM, Deterding RR (eds). *Current Diagnosis and Treatment in Pediatrics.* 18th ed. New York, NY: McGraw-Hill; 2007.

Heys SD, Park KG, Garlick PJ, et al. Nutrition and malignant disease: Implications for surgical practice. *Br J Surg.* 1992;79:614-623.

Jacobson JL, Jacobson AM. *Psychiatric Secrets.* 2nd ed. Philadelphia: Hanley and Belfus; 2001.

Kandel ER, Schwartz JH, Jessell TM (eds). *Principles of Neural Science.* 4th ed. New York, NY: McGraw-Hill; 2000.

Kaplan HI, Sadock BJ. *Synopsis of Psychiatry: Behavioral Sciences/Clinical Psychiatry.* 10th ed. Philadelphia: Lippincott Williams & Wilkins; 2007.

Katz VL, Lentz GM, Lobo RA, et al (eds). *Comprehensive Gynecology.* 5th ed. Philadelphia. PA: Mosby Elsevier; 2007.

Kliegman RM, Behrman RE, Jenson HB, Stanton BF (eds). *Nelson Textbook of Pediatrics.* 18th ed. Philadelphia, PA: WB Saunders Co.; 2007.

Lee C et al. Hepatitis B immunization for hepatitis B surface antigen positive-mothers. *Cochrane Database Syst Rev.* 2006;2:CD004790

Lee SH, Rao KCVG, Zimmerman RA (eds). *Cranial MRI and CT.* 4th ed. New York, NY: McGraw-Hill; 1999.

Mahutte NG, Duleba AJ. Evaluating diagnostic tests. http://www.utdol.com/utd/content/topic.do?topicKey=genr_med/28312&type=A&selectedTitle=1~5. Accessed 12/6/2006.

Manno EM. Subarachnoid hemorrhage. *Neurologic Clin N Am.* 2004;(22): 347-366.

Marx JA, Hockberger RS, Walls RM, et al (eds). *Rosen's Emergency Medicine Concepts and Clinical Practice.* 5th ed. St Louis, MO: Mosby; 2002.

McMillan JA, Feigin RD, DeAngelis CD, Jones MD (eds). *Oski's Pediatrics.* 4th ed. Philadelphia, PA: Lippincott Williams & Wilkins; 2006.

McPhee SJ, Lingappa VR, Ganong WF. *Pathophysiology of Disease: An Introduction to Clinical Medicine.* 5th ed. New York, NY: McGraw-Hill; 2005.

McPhee SJ, Papadakis MA, Tierney LM (eds). *Current Medical Diagnosis & Treatment.* 47th ed. New York, NY: McGraw Hill; 2008.

McQuaid KR, Isenberg JI. Medical therapy of peptic ulcer disease. *Surg Clin North Am.* 1992;72:285-316.

Meisel JL. Diagnostic approach to chest pain in adults. http://www.utdol.com/utd/content/topic.do?topicKey=pri_card/2346&type=A&selectedTitle=1~87. Accessed 12/6/2006.

Mengel MB, Schweibert LP (eds). *Family Medicine Ambulatory Care and Prevcention.* 4th ed. New York, NY: Lange Medical Books/McGraw-Hill; 2005.

Moore EE, Feliciano DV, Mattox KL. *Trauma.* 5th ed. New York, NY: McGraw-Hill; 2004.

Moore DP, Jefferson JW. *Handbook of Medical Psychiatry.* 2nd ed. Philadelphia: Mosby; 2004.

O'Brien MC. Alcoholic keotacidosis. *eMedicine Journal.* July 2007; http://www.emedicine.com/emerg/TOPIC21.HTM. Accessed May, 2008.

Patten J. *Neurological Differential Diagnosis.* 2nd ed. London: Springer-Verlag; 2001.

Rakel RE, Bope ET (eds). *Conn's Current Therapy 2006.* Philadelphia, PA: Saunders/Elsevier; 2006.

Ransom SB, Dombrowski MP, McNeeley SG, et al (eds). *Practical Strategies in Obstetrics and Gynecology.* Philadelphia, PA: WB Saunders; 2000.

Reece EA, Hobbins JC (eds). *Medicine of the Fetus and Mother.* 2nd ed. Philadelphia, PA: Lippincott; 1999.

Reilly HF, al-Kawas FH. Dieulafoy's lesion. Diagnosis and management. *Dig Dis Sci.* 1991;36:1702-1707.

Roberts JR, Hedges JR. *Clinical Procedures in Emergency Medicine.* 4th ed. Philadelphia, PA: Saunders; 2004.

Rock JA, Jones HW (eds). *TeLinde's Operative Gynecology.* 9th ed. Philadelphia, PA: Lippincott Williams & Wilkins; 2003.

Rodeck CH, Whittle MJ (eds). *Fetal Medicine: Basic Science and Clinical Practice.* London: Churchill Livingstone; 1999.

Ropper AH, Brown RH. *Adams and Victor's Principles of Neurology.* 8th ed. New York, NY: McGraw-Hill; 2005.

Rosner B. *Fundamentals of Biostatistics.* 6th ed. Pacific Grove, CA: Duxbury; 2006.

Rudolph CD, Rudolph AM, Hostetter MK, Lister G, Siegel NJ (eds). *Rudolph's Pediatrics.* 21st ed. New York, NY: McGraw-Hill; 2003.

Schwesinger WH. Is *Helicobacter pylori* a myth or the missing link? *Am J Surg.* 1996;172:411-416.

Selwyn A. Coronary artery vasospasm. *eMedicine Journal.* 2005; http://www.emedicine.com/med/topic447.htm. Accessed January 1, 2007.

South-Paul JE, Matheny SC, Lewis EL (eds). *Current Diagnosis and Treatment in Family Medicine.* 2nd ed. New York, Lange Medical Books/McGraw-Hill, 2008.

Speroff L, Glass RH, Kase NG (eds). *Clinical Gynecologic Endocrinology and Infertility.* 7th ed. Baltimore, MD: Lippincott, Williams & Wilkins; 2005.

Stenchever MA, Droegemueller W, Herbst AL, Mishell DR (eds): *Comprehensive Gynecology* 4th ed. St. Louis, Mosby, 2002.

Swaiman K, Ashwal S (eds). *Pediatric Neurology Principles and Practice.* 4th ed. Philadelphia, PA: Mosby Elsevier; 2006.

Tintinalli JE. *Emergency Medicine: A Comprehensive Study Guide.* 6th ed. New York, NY: McGraw-Hill; 2004.

Townsend CM Jr, Beauchamp RD, Evers BM, et al (eds). *Sabiston Textbook of Surgery.* 18th ed. Philadelphia, PA: Saunders; 2007.

Notes

Notes

Notes

Notes

Notes

Notes

Notes

Notes

Notes